Bones

Bones
Anorexia, OCD, and Me

Jen Dixon

To Rachel and Kyle,
for seeing past Jen II

Author's Note

Last year I tucked a draft of BONES in a drawer, convinced an unshielded depiction of my anorexia had no place on bookshelves beside the empowered women who beat their illnesses. My goal in writing was not to give advice, share what worked for me, or create a recovery journal. I wrote BONES to give an account that is rarely told from ground zero, a story that survivors only tell once they have safely escaped the clutches of anorexia and detached themselves from the creatures they became. I wanted to covey the monotonous torture of anorexia comingled with the reckless allure of bulimia and truly expose the wickedness of both. For too long, open discussion about eating disorders has been treated like abstinence-only education. If we just don't talk about them, or at least gloss over the ugly parts, they'll go away.

But mine hasn't. It moved from my childhood room into my college dorm with me. It came with me to my first day of grad school. It sat in coach with me as I flew to residential treatment, and it let me take the top bunk when I was placed on a 72-hour hold during my first year as a teacher. Anorexia is my ball-and-chain and security blanket, my worst enemy and my best friend, and my darkest yet most visible secret. OCD is its partner in crime, never quite allowing me the inner peace I need to eat.

In a dark period of compulsions and food restriction, I felt my feeble grip on recovery slip. Several social events allowed me a glimpse at an alternate universe, the life I might have had if I hadn't spent my 20s gallivanting around with my own neuroses. Anorexia is lonely yet stifling. It is the glass that separates me from the real world, simultaneously isolating and protecting me. As I get older, it becomes more and more difficult to share a "why." Why do I take comfort in what will most likely kill me?

There's an often-repeated cliché that eating disorders aren't about the food, but what does that mean? It's a true statement, but its lack of specificity has always bothered me. After many daydreams of what it would be like to just be honest for once after a lifetime of secrets, to explain bluntly why it's not as simple as "just eat," I began to write. I started in the middle, dancing around the sore spots as I'm adept at doing. Filling blank pages with the black and white truth made it more real, and many days I feared my own words would crawl into bed with me later that night. But I needed for once in my life to be candid, even if it was just confessing to an empty page.

During a tide of mental health awareness movements, I still felt lost at sea. I wondered how many people out there were like me. My intention was not to release a self-help book or to glamorize a disease when there is no glamor to be found. I didn't know if I deserved to write an account of my illness when I was still in the midst of recovery. But I wrote anyways, hoping an unfiltered account of my experience would make you laugh when you shouldn't, understand the incomprehensible, and stay awake a few extra minutes at night turning the pages of my life.

Fashion Killa

"Fuck you all. I hate this fucking family! I'm not coming back." This is one of my earliest childhood memories. My mom standing in the doorway of the laundry room, brown leather purse in hand, voice trembling with rage and desperation. Desperation to not be my mom any more. Infantile amnesia has obscured my ability to recall my fifth birthday party at Skate Station, our family trip to the Rocky Mountains the summer I turned six, or the cooler my parents filled with orange wedges each week to bring to my soccer games. Unfortunately, this is the pivotal moment burned in my memory, followed by the sound of the garage door opening and the screech of tires as my mom barrels down the driveway to free herself from her suburban ensnarement.

The lead-up to this monumental scene is an afternoon spent at the Sweetwater Mall, a small-town shopping center filled with the aroma of Auntie Ann's pretzels and hormonal teenage boys doused in cologne, ready to fall on the latest trend. My sister and I flank my mom as we walk past the over-perfumed Clinique ladies with foundation-coated cheeks two shades too dark. It's the summer before kindergarten, and it's time for me to pick out a dress to wear to Grandaddy's 70th birthday.

It's taken a certain degree of bribery to get me here. Mom has promised if I suffer through this torturous process and successfully choose a form-fitting dress, if I soldier through an afternoon in the JCPenney Kids Department, we can stop by the cigar shop on our way out. I do not want a cigar. I'm five years old and this is not that kind of memoir. But this particular shop, Smoke-n-Snuff, has an assortment of ceramic model dogs in the display window. They beg me to bring them home, and I can hear their whimpers through the glass. I'm mesmerized every time we walk by, tugging my mom to stop walking as I let go of her hand.

Natalie is tall and gangly, a walking scarecrow with stringy brown hair, oversized coke bottle glasses, and denim shorts that settle somewhere between her hips and armpits. She will remain homely for the next five years, until puberty turns her into a swan. But she's my older sister, and to me she is perfect.

I'm a short, stocky tomboy walking the fine line between sporty and is-she-going-to-be-a-lesbian? I spend my days playing basketball, digging holes to China, and indulging in other pastimes of a child in an idyllic 90s sitcom. This trip to the mall is an interruption, and I feel as comfortable in a dress as a little boy would. I hate that I'm not supposed to sit with my legs splayed, and even more so hate the prospect of spending an entire day feeling the cotton fabric cling to my body, never letting me escape the tactile reminder that my stomach does not lie flat like Natalie's.

Mom loves to blow raspberries into my belly button. She finds my tummy adorable. I feel more comfortable in oversized T-shirts and shorts that nearly fall off, allowing me to forget my tragic flaw. Overall, I'm a well-adjusted child, constantly giggling, making up silly songs, and freezing my parents' underwear. But shopping is my Achilles heel. The way the different fabrics cling, how I look in the dressing room mirrors, and the fact that Natalie never looks like she is about to spill out of her own skin, all make me want to teleport myself out of the mall and arrive in any place or time other than here.

After four hours of trying on every dress in my size, I hate the way every last one feels. I tug at the fabric, trying to find a position where it doesn't stick to my stomach. But no matter which way I pull, nothing feels right. I throw a temper tantrum, tears flowing down my cheeks as I look in the mirror of JCPenney. My tummy resembles a beach ball that needs more space, something much larger. This lacy abomination is two sizes too tight for my comfort and a size too loose for my mom's.

In a sharp whisper she tells me, "Shut up. You're making a scene. We're going home, just put your clothes back on." She grabs my hand, her purse, and my sister and sweeps us back to her minivan, defeated.

She buckles me into the captain's seat next to my sister as I clench my calf muscles until they cramp, crying and pouting that nothing felt right. As she turns the key in the ignition, Carol King picks up where she left off and Mom begins to cry with me, or more accurately at me, as we begin our journey home. My sister, eight years old and the most mature one in the car, looks out the window, waiting to get away from this minivan of mental illness. We get home, Mom shuts herself in her bedroom, and Dad helps Natalie and me brush our teeth for bed.

I throw on my favorite Barney T-shirt, soft and loose, and Mom tells me to put on a pair of silk pajamas from the Limited Too. They had been an unwelcome gift under the Christmas tree last year, the cheerful multicolored stars disguising the cruelty of the elastic waistband that dug into my fat rolls and squeezed me like a noose. All I can hear when I wear those shorts is *You're fat. You're fat. You're fat.*

"You're being a brat. Put them on. Put the damn pajamas on!" Mom rarely curses, but she's losing her patience.

"Debbie, just let her wear what she wants. It's been a long day and it's not a big deal," Dad says, attempting to de-escalate. Contradicting my mom is a rare occurrence for him, soon to become more seldom.

My sister chimes in, likely more out of jealousy than support. I receive a disproportionate amount of attention, and she is the honorary middle child. "You're always so focused on Jen. Why does it matter what she wears to bed? Just stop picking at every little thing."

It's true. I'm my mom's fixer-upper, her pet project, the identified patient in the family.

Voices escalate. This is no longer my battle. Even at five years old I realize this. It will be a very long time before my dad is able to get himself out of this one.

The tension reaches the climax when my mom screams, "Fuck you all. I hate this fucking family! I'm not coming back." And with a definitive slam of the laundry room door, it's now just the three of us.

My dad remains calm. "It's okay girls, she'll be back. Let's get you tucked in."

I waste no time, eager to take advantage of the profanity situation. "Fuck. Fuck shuck. Fuck yuck duck."

"Jenna Dixon, if you say that word one more time you won't play with your dog collection for a year." I look at my 200 model dogs, mostly plastic but a few ceramic, and realize they need me to control my tongue.

"Is Mom going to come back?" I ask. He assures me that of course she will, that she loves us all very much and that even grown-ups need to cool off sometimes.

I try to mask my disappointment. Dad uses real butter on our grilled cheese bagels, doesn't make us do as many chores, and never screams when he's upset. He lets me come with him when he needs to go to the landfill, and he uses his environmental engineering skills to tell me how long it will take various scraps to decompose. He tells the best bedtime stories, concocted with no preparation; sagas of Ghostie Bobo and Princess Alaba getting caught in elevators full of water balloons.

At the same time, the whole fiasco is my fault, and I don't want to carry my mom's permanent departure on my conscience for the rest of my life. Deep down I feel uneasy, like something permanent and awful has just happened and life will never be the same.

The next morning, I wake up to the moan of the garage door opening. I lie in bed and listen intently, not wanting to let my model dogs know I'm awake. Did I just hear a faint barking, a pitter patter of ceramic paws against my wooden shelves? The smell of hazelnut coffee wafts under my door, so I slip out of the covers and enter the kitchen. My mom is sitting at the table, her mournful eyes and shaky voice leaving no question that she is wounded. I'm familiar with this face and my stomach sinks to my toes. A cloud of misery will linger over the dinner table for days to remind my dad of his perceived transgressions.

There's a balled-up tissue next to her hand and the *Sanford Sun* spread out on the kitchen table. I feel a pang of guilt for my slight disappointment that she's back and try to stuff the emotion back down. The newspaper is open to the Real Estate section. At five, I don't yet know that this is the first of many empty threats she'll make about leaving.

"I'm a horrible mother." "You would be better off without me." "You don't love me." These will become familiar, empty words. I don't know that several days later, she will move her things back into the master bedroom and carry on with life as if the past week never happened at all. She will transform back into the mother that makes up silly songs as our whole family cuddles in front of *The Sound of Music*, surprises us after school with stickers and movie tickets to *The Lion King*, or takes us to mother-daughter read-alouds of *Ramona* at the public library.

"We need to talk about last night," she says to me as I approach the breakfast table, amplifying the shakiness in her voice. I immediately burst into tears, never able to regulate my emotions separately from hers. My sister casually pours herself a glass of orange juice, the sound of her gulps drowning out my snivels.

"Natalie, do you even care that I'm upset? Do you want me to leave again?"

Natalie looks at my mother and shakes her head no, but she doesn't exert herself.

I don't remember what words were exchanged during the next twenty minutes of rehashing. All I remember is an errant hair on my mom's left shoulder, right above the purple rose on her nightgown. It's limp and resembles a lost letter C. My own tears stop and I focus on the white follicle at the end of the hair. *What if it gets on me? What if it falls into her bowl, sinks to the bottom of the blue-tinged skim milk, and slides down her throat as she brings the bowl to her lips?* I feel my own throat contract as I stifle a gag. I go to the sink, douse my hands with lemon dish soap, and scrub with vigor.

"Honey, come over here and give me a hug. Mommy is sorry we had a fight. I'm not going to leave."

This whole explosion was my fault, my own temper tantrum, my own inability to regulate my emotions, and all I can focus on is not getting the hair on me. I try not to flinch as she pulls me close to her chest.

It frustrates me that there isn't a bigger spark, a bigger inciting event for when my problems began. I've spent years searching for a "why." Why am I drawn to self-sabotage? How justified am I to resent a mother who is no more complicated than I am? Have I repressed some horrific trauma? The most puzzling thing for me is that I don't have an alcoholic father who left welts on my back or a sadistic rapist that popped out of the bushes to steal my childhood. The lack of one extreme event triggering my OCD and anorexia means the issue lies within me, and the shame I carry with this knowledge has led to years of minimizing the issue and feeling I don't deserve to be as sick as I am.

Lord Give Me A Sign (Munchkin Remix)

Immediately after the fight with my mom, I begin washing my hands every time she kisses me. I can see the disappointment in her eyes as she tucks me in and plants kisses on my chubby cheeks and cherub tummy. I scramble out of bed and wash my hands, perturbed by the contamination.

"Jen, why don't you do that when Dad kisses you?" She isn't accusatory, just hurt.

Dad has short hair, and it doesn't fall out to rest on his shoulders. It doesn't find its way onto the breakfast table to cling to the sweat from a glass of milk. I don't want to hurt her. I need to wash my hands after her kisses, but I can find a way to compensate and make it right with the universe.

In my first weeks of kindergarten, Ms. Thatcher scolds me for not walking in a straight line to the lunchroom. "Jen, you need to be walking right behind Nicolas. Pretend he's leaving footprints in the sand and you are trying to step in them."

Ms. Thatcher doesn't understand that I'm saving my mom's back. Along with Ms. Mary Mack All Dressed in Black, we chant "Step on a Crack, Break Your Mother's Back" as we jump rope at recess.

I can't even say it out loud. I feel guilty for letting the mantra enter my ears, and I try to hum it away, try to push the chorus out of my eardrums so the words can't enter. But they do, and since I've heard them, I too am complicit. I avoid cracks in the sidewalk, stutter stepping when necessary to adjust my path. My concern for my mother's back instantly subsides, and I'm encouraged that my strategy is working.

Soon thereafter, I take note of the alternating white and teal pattern of the tiles at school. The seams around each tile are technically cracks. God speaks to me. I need to stop stepping on the seams between these tiles as well. At first, my parents think this is an endearing habit, smiling as they see me hop from tile to tile in the drugstore. Luckily, when I hold my mother's hand, I give her immunity and no longer have to take these precautions.

God speaks to me again several weeks later as I'm once again failing to step into Nicolas' footprints on the way to lunch. I'm surprised that God had selected me as His Chosen One. My parents are not devout by any means. My mother was raised in a stiflingly religious Church of Christ, and my father was a lifelong agnostic. But God spoke to Mary and told her a child would be born. Now he is speaking to me and telling me there are lives that most people aren't aware of, and it is my duty to listen.

Jen, every time you take a step you are crushing a munchkin, He tells me.

I imagine the Oompa Loompas in *Charlie and the Chocolate Factory*, but small enough to fit in my hand, with denim jeans, suspenders, and solid primary colored shirts.

You can't see them but they are everywhere. They don't just live in the sidewalk cracks and the perimeter of the tiles. They also live in every teal tile at school, and under the floor at home. They can be anywhere. No matter what you do, you'll end up stepping on them and crushing them, God warns.

This is an enormous responsibility. God has spoken. I realize that every time I step down, I kill countless adorable micro-humans. But God has already realized there is no way to avoid stepping down, so he offers a solution, which I later learn is a compulsion. The munchkins are inflatable, so I can save them if I act quickly. Every ninth step I take I must scoop my hand along the ground so I can pick up any victims I've crushed, curl my hand around the deflated bodies, and blow life back into them. If I wait too long, they will stay forever deflated, never to live out their munchkin lives with munchkin families and munchkin puppies.

God's voice sounds suspiciously similar to my own thoughts. But I would be a monster to not put in the minimal effort to blow into my hand. It's such a simple gesture, especially if it means saving thousands of innocent lives.

I try to hide what I'm doing. I avert my eyes as I puff into my hand and feel my cheeks flush when I think I've been seen. I can't see the munchkins or hear their squeals, but in church they say to have faith. In my gut I'm skeptical. Maybe this is not actually God. But the one percent chance I could be wrong keeps me going.

The habit is exhausting. I have to count my steps, and after a few weeks there is no longer immunity for holding my mom's hand. She notices I dart in different directions and avoid tiles when we run errands together, following rules to a game only I know exists. I try to evade detection as I inflate the pint-sized victims, but it gets harder to hide. Sometimes there's no covert way to rescue them, and I make a mental note to atone for it later in the privacy of my bedroom. I blow extra air into my palm and let it float down the sidewalk of our suburban neighborhood in search of the munchkin I left dying on the operating table as I went down the playground slide.

For weeks I strictly adhere to God's instructions, until I begin to question His authority. I still don't see any munchkins, and whenever I consider telling my sister, I know she will laugh at me. God reminds me that some of the munchkins are pregnant. Some of them get their feelings hurt very easily, and others have pet puppies that squeal and whimper in pain every time I step on their tails and sever their warm, wriggly bodies.

I start to doubt myself, replaying my day in my head. *Did I forget to blow at recess today? Did I blow hard enough to reinflate in Eckerds Pharmacy?* I picture Mary Munchkin writhing in pain on the floor, crushed under the weight of my jelly sandals. Sitting in a chair becomes difficult. There are four legs, meaning four munchkins to reinflate. Plus, the legs drag on the ground as I pull it away from the table, dismembering munchkins like a snow plow. I try to cut up a pork tenderloin and focus on my sister's summary of her guitar lesson, but all I can hear are the imaginary screams of a munchkin genocide beneath the table.

I took life very seriously as a child. The awesome responsibility of needing to stop every potential hazard that popped into my mind during naptime at school, or being solely responsible for teaching the family cat to read, saddled me down. I sometimes wondered if Natalie too stared into the darkness after she was tucked into bed, realizing that in one catastrophic event, the whole universe could end and we would cease to exist like modern-day dinosaurs.

In hindsight, I do not think Natalie worried about mass extinctions. To this day, she functions off of logic, rarely crying or getting angry. Explosive temper must be a recessive trait for her, a force that lies deep within but is overshadowed by the calm and measured mannerisms of my dad.

We play tag inside the house one October afternoon, too cold to go outside, and the game is so much fun I inadvertently run over an entire community of munchkins. Realizing my carelessness and performing CPR, Natalie catches me in the act. She gets very close and speaks in a hushed voice, a detective ready to crack the case.

"Why do you keep puffing into your hands? Every time I look at you, you're blowing into your hands like a weirdo." Her voice is not accusatory. She seems genuinely curious and amused, the corners of her mouth curled into a smile.

A lump forms in my throat. It's been such a heavy weight to carry. "Do you promise you won't tell Mom and Dad?" I whisper.

"I won't tell them if you tell me right now. But if you don't, I'm going to tell Mom to ask you herself." Her voice drips in superiority.

It's hard for me to spit it out, to let my secret mission exist somewhere outside of my own head. I pull at the skin beneath my chin and tug it down until it hangs as low as Grammy's gobbler. I scratch at my neck and the feeling of nails in flesh momentarily lifts me out of this humiliation.

"God told me that there's..." I can't say the words without giggling. I thought that I would cry but I don't. The weight of the last months propulses out of my body in uncontrollable laughter. I cannot hold in my secret or censor it for the ears of The Unchosen. "There are munchkins that I crush every time I step on them. The only way to save them is to blow into my hand. I know it sounds crazy, but God told me that I'm not crazy and I'm saving their lives. Everywhere you walk you're crushing them, but God picked me to save them. Please don't tell Mom and Dad."

Within the hour I learn that Natalie is a colossal snitch. My parents, convinced their daughter has a prodigious case of schizophrenia at the tender age of five, book a session with Les Krause. Dr. Krause is in her mid-forties with a modified mullet that could pass as blonde but is at least half gray, and thick glasses that remind me of goggles. At the end of every session, I get to pick a toy from her treasure chest and play in the waiting room while she talks to my mom.

I look forward to seeing her mostly because of the toy, but also because it feels good to have somebody take the weight of the munchkin world off my shoulders and share it with me. But trusting Dr. Krause is an enormous risk. Her dowdy appearance makes it even more shocking that she is a gambler, willing to take the chance and assume that God is not speaking to me.

"Does the voice sound like God or more like a voice inside of your head?" she asks me during our first meeting. I had always thought it strange that God sounded like a little girl. "Can you actually see the munchkins or is the voice just telling you they're there?"

I had visualized the munchkins in my imagination, vividly dancing around in their denim jeans. But I had never actually seen them with my own two eyes.

"What you're hearing are thoughts coming from your own brain, Jen, not God. If you listen to them and act on them, they'll get louder. The only way to stop them is to not do what they want you to. At first they'll get louder than ever, but eventually they'll become so quiet you can't hear them anymore."

In terminology that I cannot understand, while I teach a plastic dog his times tables in the waiting room, Dr. Krause explains to my parents that I'm not schizophrenic. I'm displaying early signs of obsessive compulsive disorder, where a tiny seed of doubt in my brain will be enough for me to do everything in my power to make it go away. Some sufferers might check locks for three hours, eventually loosening the door handle beyond repair; or wash their hands until they bleed just in case there's a germ; or be late for work to turn around just one more time to check the coffee pot. I don't know for certain if these are the specific examples she used with my parents, but these events will later become my own experience.

She explains to them that the difference between my disorder and insanity is that I know that my thoughts are not rational, so I try to hide my compulsions out of embarrassment. I will have a brief dance with insanity much later in life, but at this point my diagnosis is a colossal relief.

I leave my weekly therapy sessions with calves that are sore from clenching, shirts missing buttons from nervous tugging, and eyes puffy from frustrated tears.

"We're going to do exactly what your OCD is telling you not to," Dr. Krause explains. We're going to disobey God and perform sacrilegious exercises in the middle of the day, the sun shining cheerfully on a potential murder scene.

"We're going to go one step at a time. Just inside this office. I'll do it with you, Jen. We're going to stomp. And then we'll both sit on our hands and not blow on them, even if we really want to." Dr. Krause's clogs coax me to join her, and soon my high tops are crushing munchkins I now realize don't exist.

Weeks pass and things get easier. I'm stepping in Nicolas's footprints on the way to the cafeteria. I'm pulling out my dinner chair and instinctively sitting on my hands. I make a miraculous recovery, and within a few months the munchkins are gone and so is God's voice. My parents are amazed at this new cutting-edge treatment, exposure therapy, that has turned their schizophrenic daughter into a happy little girl again.

No medication is prescribed, and Dr. Krause tells us it may have been a response to a stressful event. I have been instructed not to tell Dr. Krause about the very trashy Fuck You Fight, so she is being hypothetical. But if one event did trigger the munchkins, now that it's over I may never experience another flare-up. Or it might be an issue in my brain that predisposes me to anxiety. It might not have been caused by one specific incident at all, and in that case the symptoms might come back.

The seed has been planted in my parents' minds. I am the problem child. Not in a bad way. But my mom's concerns that I'm different have been validated, and her guilt that the explosive fight may have been the root cause never leaves her mind. I'm a bit more fragile, a bit more delicate than my sister. God's voice is gone, but will it return? I will need extra attention, extra observations from my mom to prevent a relapse into MunchkinLand and to keep me on the path to normalcy.

Unfortunately, my mom's unease was partially correct. Obsessive compulsive disorder is a brain disorder. It wasn't a quirky thought that randomly hit me, and it wasn't the munchkins I needed to get rid of. It was the constant need to check, to erase any doubt or uncertainty from my life. Unfortunately, this need had not been stomped out with the munchkins.

Fireman

The next few years were full of normal childhood memories. Family vacations, basketball trophies, and slumber parties were on the surface. But underneath the brightness, I was hiding one all-encompassing, hyper-focused obsession after another.

In first grade, two important men from the Linnea County Fire Department visit my class to go over fire safety. I learn it's up to me and you and everybody to prevent housefires. I realize that I have not been doing my part. Mom keeps her to-do list right next to the stove, an 8.5x14 inch yellow legal pad. Next to it is a thick stack of clipped coupons, the different sizes never neatly aligning. All of this is a blatant fire hazard my mom is oblivious to because she did not hear the guest speakers.

It's my responsibility to educate her that she's unwittingly jeopardizing our home and every home in our neighborhood, and that inevitably our golden retriever's bushy tail will become a roasting stick. Buddy will end up a charred clump of ashes. I have been warned and it is now my duty to save our beloved Buddy, all of my model dogs, and every dog (and human, I suppose) in our neighborhood.

Mom refuses to move her work station, insistent that a stove that is off cannot catch fire. I'm forced to work around her negligence. Every night I pack a fire suitcase before going to bed. I must cross-check each of my 362 model dogs with an attendance sheet I keep in a manilla folder labeled **Dog Family Roster**. The businesslike words do not match my failed depictions of puppies scribbled in clumsy crayon and my attempts at motivational phrases such as **Dogs Rule!** If I forget to check one dog off the attendance sheet, I have to start from the beginning to ensure none of them get left behind to burn in the flames. My parents wonder if maybe we should visit Dr. Krause again for exposure therapy, but what is she going to do this time, light me on fire?

After I'm put to bed at night a new universe emerges, one that is free from any outside observations. Over the years, the universe I'm submerged in changes, but it is always my arena, where the rules that make perfect sense to me are no longer under the scrutiny of outsiders.

In sixth grade it's the gnats. I fill the gap under my door with a beach towel to block the light from streaming underneath, so as not to tip off my parents that I am still awake. I then set my black rolly desk chair on my bed (in hindsight an accident waiting to happen) and stand on it for hours waiting to see if a gnat might be drawn to the light. It is as satisfying as popping a pimple, but when I want to stop and go to bed it's an itch I have to scratch.

I should go to bed. But if I give up now and turn the lights out, I might miss the next gnat by mere seconds. Just one more minute. One more gnat.

I lost a lot of sleep that year.

Ms. Moon is my Language Arts teacher, a petite woman with close-cropped black curls. She's new to middle school after years of teaching second grade at a private religious school. Her class is insultingly easy, as if she took the second grade syllabus, erased any reference to God or Jesus, and recycled every lesson. I sit next to a girl who smells like pee, my only true memory from this particular course other than the stuffed Tweety Bird at the front of the room, scandalously naked.

Nobody pees in their pants every day. And if you did it wouldn't smell for a while. Wet pee doesn't smell very much, it would have to dry. So is there dried pee on her clothes? She wears different clothes every day. Maybe someone pees in her hair? Could the scent stick to me? Do I smell like pee after this class and not know it?

The rest of my focus, though, is on Ms. Moon's classroom plant. It's an elephant ear with succulent green leaves growing from a terracotta pot adorned with red and blue polka dots. With the approximate frequency of once a week, I see a tiny black speck, smaller than the ones on my ceiling at home, fly out from the soil of the plant. Its body contrasts with the white cinder block walls. It must be chasing the scent of urine. It's a rare opportunity, but nothing feels so satisfying as smooshing these specks against the wall with my index finger and brushing the bodies onto the thin blue commercial rug.

"Jen, look up here. Did you write that down?" Ms. Moon is very gentle, never one to yell or scold. Through the adult lens of being a teacher, I'm sure she was kindly telling me to fucking pay attention. Eventually it becomes clear I cannot thrive in this environment, much like the gnats.

"Jen, I'm going to move you closer to the front today, away from whatever is so interesting about that wall." It's difficult to explain, but this is a relief. The gnats were a terrible mixture of fascination and total inability to restrain myself from compulsively seeking them out.

I never make less than an A, but I'm insecure about my intelligence. I struggle more with homework than Natalie, likely because I'm focused on gnats and urine in the classroom. Natalie finishes her assignments before dinner every night, and I take longer, shed more tears, and break more pencil tips as I stab them with frustration into the seams of my textbooks. I'm not as smart as she is and I need to try harder. I need to put in extra work to earn my A's.

After my parents tuck me in, I take my lamp off the freshly polished glass of my bedside table and pull my backpack into my closet, shoving aside the rarely used dress sandals that clutter the floor. I cross-reference each syllabus and ensure every paper in all six binders is in perfect order. Then I repeat the process over and over again until it feels right.

It can't be that simple though. I've been told that middle school is the real deal, so I begin to label every worksheet with my own secret code, a combination of randomized letters and numbers. I now refer to the math worksheet with circus animals around the border, patronizingly disguising the seriousness of its content, as **Form AX21L**. This way I can write the form number in my planner and add an extra layer to my checking system. This will make it nearly impossible to forget an assignment. It sounds simple enough. But with six classes and multiple assignments a day, I drown with the nightly burden of organizing my school work, let alone actually doing what was assigned.

I rarely struggle to understand concepts in class, but the details drive me insane. I'm aware that I ask too many questions of teachers and I'm self-conscious about it.

"Do you want the heading to say period 'Three' or period '3?' Will you take off points if I don't skip a line? Should I write my middle name or just my first and last?" I hate that I ask these types of nitpicky questions, but I can't relax until I do.

One staple please! is a frequent reminder in red ink on my returned assignments, referring to the eyesore of the twelve staples I considered barely adequate. As a teacher now, I can easily identify the students with anxiety issues. The questions are never about content, always about minutiae, and frankly, extremely fucking annoying.

My teachers tell my parents that I am exhibiting signs of anxiety. Soon thereafter, I return to Dr. Krause for a tune-up. This time there are no munchkins to stomp out. It's not as simple as setting my chair down over and over again. Exposure therapy now consists of playing tug of war with my dad each night as he attempts to pry my backpack out of my hands as my white knuckles clutch the straps and I scream in protest.

"I'm not done yet! I'm not done yet!" I wail as I beg for five more minutes.

Doctor Krause recommends medication. So after school one day I'm introduced to Dr. Starkist, a burly Armenian psychiatrist. He has a bushy black beard that covers most of his face and a permanent twinkle in his eyes as if he and I share a secret that only he is aware of. I like him. He's comfortable with silence and never fills emptiness with senseless words as he observes my mother and me. He doesn't want to hear about my disorder at first. He is interested in my classes, whether I like the other girls on my basketball team, and how old Buddy is.

Mom is impatient, wanting to discuss what we're here for. "The nightly fits are horrible, and the whole family is exhausted. I volunteer in the front office of her school, and some days her teachers tell me that she isn't able to focus, digging through her backpack instead of listening. We're very involved parents and we just want her to be successful. I also wanted to talk about age appropriate behavior. She doesn't seem interested in boys and she goes to school with wet hair and no makeup. She's eating more than usual, probably because of all the stress, and she doesn't play outside anymore. All she does is homework. When she was a child she used to be fascinated by prostitutes. We once caught her looking up pictures of penises on the family computer. Penis.com. She talks my ear off some days, very hyper."

The clock sitting atop his desk ticks. He looks amused as he studies my mother, his eyes settling on the yellow legal pad sitting in her lap, a list of concerns two pages in length.

"This is part of the problem." There's no judgement in his voice.

Dr. Starkist does not know the Debbie Rules. Other than panic disorder, there's no diagnosis I can use to describe my mom, other than she is clinically sensitive to any criticism and will hold onto it for weeks, making everyone around her miserable. Two decades later, she can't remember my dog's name on my weekly visits, but she can hold onto a perceived slight as if her Alzheimer's is nothing more than an overhyped case of the sniffles.

"We're not going to see Dr. Starkist anymore. He's a total jerk. That was unbelievable. He probably graduated last in his med school," she says later that evening at the dinner table as she vents to my father.

Unfortunately, this is a small city and Dr. Starkist is the only pediatric psychiatrist my dad's insurance will pay for. For all future appointments, she suffers in silence until we reach the car and she can fume about this "incompetent, obese bastard."

I'm put on Prozac and Concerta and am officially diagnosed with obsessive compulsive disorder and ADHD. I think they threw the latter diagnosis in there because it was the 90s, and if you were under twelve and breathing, you had ADHD.

Over the years I will come on and off of various medications. Buspar, clonazepam, diazepam, Lexapro, Paxil, Prozac, Remeron, Rexulti, Strattera, and various other cocktails. This, along with the occasional Xanax my mom will share, force on me actually, when I won't stop screaming about locked doors or unfinished dissertations on the anatomy of an insect.

One day, as we check out of an appointment with Dr. Starkist, his nurse casually mentions to my mother that because antidepressants can lead to weight gain, it's a good idea to keep an eye out for an increase in appetite.

Fatty Girl

My mom is my best friend. I love coming home from school and telling her about my day; what boy I have a crush on, which teacher yelled at a troublemaker, and whether or not Mr. Hamilton combed his overgrown eyebrows. She listens to all of my babble, helps me hatch plans to lure in my crush, and guides me toward nice friends. It would be easy to portray her as a villain in my story, but she isn't. She's a damn good mom. Our relationship is just complicated.

In the spring of my sixth grade year, my friend Olivia turns twelve and I attend her birthday party. My crush is there and we play ping pong. I carry Olivia's little cairn terrier around all night, dancing to *Who Let the Dogs Out* and *Mambo No. 5* while I swing him around. We swim in her peanut-shaped pool until the boys start pelting water balloons at us. When I get home,

I am recounting these details to my mom when she interrupts me to ask, "What did you eat for dinner?"

That was one of the best parts. Olivia's parents ordered Papa John's and a cookie cake, and there was enough food for me to snag three pieces of pizza and two pieces of cake, including a corner piece. Mom must not have heard me, because she isn't excited.

"Honey, I've been meaning to talk to you. That's a lot of food. I think the Prozac is making you hungrier, and with how stressed out you've been, you're getting chubby. Especially around the tummy area."

"I'm not chubby," I say, bristling at the accusation.

"You're still a beautiful girl, by far prettier than any one of your friends. But we need to watch your weight more than the other girls because of the Prozac."

I instinctively pull my pool towel over my stomach, hoping the flab will go away if I can't see it. I tug on a clump of chlorine-coated hair and crunch it between my fingers. She's wrong. I remind myself that I can do ten chin ups and run faster than anyone in my class. I'm not chubby. I don't come from the sort of family where the kids are chubby.

I finish my sixth grade year focused on getting straight As, hoping my crush will ask me to the next after-school dance, and vying for a spot in the popular crew. I cover up my baby fat with fashionable matching sets from the Limited Too, but two sizes too large.

The first week of summer, my friend Hannah, one of the most popular girls in school, invites me to her family beach house. Hannah's parents are newly divorced, and the beach house is a consolation prize her dad won in the settlement. Hannah has a moon face and freckles, and a way of making her opinions seem undeniably correct. Her older brother is in college and knows things, and this gives her copious amounts of credibility.

On the first day of our vacation, having just pretended to put on sunscreen, I walk on to her wooden deck overlooking the shoreline. I'm ready to play in the water and boogie board for the rest of the afternoon. But as I climb down the steps to walk toward the sand dunes, Hannah asks, "Do you know what you have?"

I don't know how, but I instinctively know what she's about to say. She's going to comment on the weight I've put on. Before she can answer her own question, I reflexively cross my arms over my stomach.

Please don't say I'm fat. Please don't say I'm fat. Please don't say I'm fat.

"You have love handles." She says it as if she's telling me I have brown hair.

"I know. I'm planning on losing weight this summer," I reply nonchalantly, as if getting love handles was part of my plan.

The next morning I keep true to my word. Now that school is out I can focus fully on a new mission, which is to take care of all the Prozac weight that has crept up on me. Every day for the rest of the summer, I run a three mile loop when I wake up, perform 300 crunches in front of *The Brady Bunch*, and execute fifty pushups with admittedly poor form. I start a dog walking service, plastering clipart all over a flyer I design myself, and tape one to every mailbox within biking distance. I'm a young entrepreneur on a scooter, saving up money for vet school and burning calories simultaneously.

I adjust my diet to be modeled after my mom's. Mom is a slender woman and her diet is low-fat, with lots of vegetables and fruit. At dinner, if I do not eat more than her, I assume I'm not overeating. My plan is wildly successful, and unlike cross-referencing math worksheets with my planner, which only annoyed my parents and teachers, now other mothers fawn over me at pool parties and friends marvel at how much I've changed in one summer. My baby fat is gone.

"Jen, you've lost so much weight." "You're shooting up." "I saw you running yesterday and you were going so fast. I could never be that disciplined!" These comments are gasoline in my tank, fueling me to keep going.

By August, Mom tells me I've lost enough weight. "You could actually put on a few pounds, honey. I bought you some of that ice cream you love, Moose Tracks. Tomato soup is healthy, but it may not be enough to replace everything you burn off running so much."

But she's not going to take this away from me. I've finally found something I'm good at and it supplants every other obsession that creeps into my mind. I've found my passion and I'm never letting go.

***

The smell of fifty seventh graders, half of whom have yet to discover deodorant, wafts through the bleachers of the gymnasium in my first week back to school. Coach Pell calls my name and I step on the scale. She starts at 96, my weight at the end of last year. She slides the black counterbalance to the left until it clicks in place at 90. Not yet. She slides it further to the left until I hear it clink into 80. Still too high. Her eyes widen as it stops at 70, just a smidge too low. The beam finally balances at 73.

"Girl, how did you lose 23 pounds in three months?" she asks, a mixture of impressed and concerned.

"I've been running!" I tell her, beaming.

Dr. Krause warns my parents that OCD and eating disorders often coexist, and I am more at risk for developing one.

"That's a little dramatic," Mom tells me on the ride home. "Dr. Krause told me she drinks whole milk and uses full fat butter. I don't think she understands this whole running thing. She's good at what she does, but she doesn't know much about nutrition. We live a very healthy lifestyle that people who sit in front of the TV all day don't understand."

My running is a convenient excuse to justify my weight loss. I'm not aware it's an excuse. I just know I'm running to burn calories, but I'm also winning lots of local races. I lose interest in fitting in with the popular girls and make excuses to miss the pool parties where pizza and cake are waiting to sweep me back to the chlorine-drenched glutton I was less than a year ago.

My world revolves around running. For my thirteenth birthday my parents give me a gym membership and I discover that building muscle makes me look even more like the models on the cover of *Men's Fitness*, invincibly staring at the camera with bulging biceps and shredded six-packs. With strict dieting, running, and lifting weights, I finally start to see what I've wished for my whole life. By Christmas of my seventh grade year, six small squares appear on my stomach. I finally have a six-pack, the furthest possible extreme from the little girl in the dressing room clenching her fists and crying as she tried on dresses. Some days at school, I raise my hand to go to the bathroom only to stand in the handicap stall and lift up my shirt, making sure the lines carved in my stomach have not faded during the school day.

The munchkins are gone. I'm making straight As with half of the effort. I'm more interested in doing crunches than killing gnats. My life has never been better and I have finally conquered OCD.

Blood On My Hands

I didn't want to call Angela. My mom was tired of me watching Lifetime movies alone, chipping away at Thomas Kinkade jigsaw puzzles on the floor of my parents' bedroom every weekend. I've never struggled to make friends but feel more content in the company of my own thoughts. After so many years, it's difficult for me to know whether my introversion is a result of my eating disorder or just my nature. But summer training has begun for the high school cross country team, and my mom wants to make sure I begin ninth grade with a good group of friends.

Briefly before meeting my dad, my mom was a secretary for a young Korean accountant named Andrew Kim. Mr. Kim is a tiny, chipper man sporting a fanny pack I can only assume is full of dad jokes. He's an unapologetically corny corporate hotshot. His wife is an account executive at a local advertising agency and a self-described workaholic. Angela is their middle daughter, a sporty, piano-playing honor roll student who has an affinity for *Harry Potter* and falls on every single trail run our team goes on.

Angela is a year and a half older than me, and I cringe at the idea of making the first move. Why would she want to hang out with a freshman? I squint my eyes as I punch in her phone number and let my finger hover over the green button for several seconds. I'm more nervous than happy when she agrees to meet at Royal Cinema the following Friday to see *Pirates of the Caribbean*. I find the movie incredibly confusing, mostly because I spend the whole time wondering if Angela is having fun or just being nice because our parents used to work together.

But she wasn't just being nice. Before I get into my dad's minivan to drive home, she invites me over the next day so we can do our long run together. Walking up her drive in the light of day, the first thing I notice is that her house looks like the houses in *The Wonder Years*. Large two-story homes with two car garages sit right beside 1500 square foot fixer-uppers with bench presses in the front yard. The hopscotch outlines in the street and tricycles in the driveways hint that families fill these homes. I ring the doorbell.

When I have friends over there is lots of preparation. We vacuum the house, mop the floors, and light scented candles to let them know that I come from a good home. My mom usually bakes something and greets them at the door with a warm southern smile. I stand on the Kims' front porch for a full five minutes before I dare ring the doorbell again, and after another extended wait, I infer it is broken. I knock and Mrs. Kim answers. She gives me a brief greeting before returning to her preparations for a work conference. The house isn't dirty but it isn't clean.

Angela gives me a tour and I'm in awe. She has all of the cool gadgets a high school girl longs for, from gravity-defying Moon Boots to bounce around the house in to her own personal mini-fridge stocked with Diet Coke. Her door is plastered with magazine cutouts of Josh Hartnett, Britney Spears, and Shakira. There's shag carpet in her bathroom, which I'll soon learn is poor design when she absentmindedly forgets she has drawn a bath and floods the entire bathroom. Her mom's reaction indicates this is a frequent occurrence.

What I don't know at the time is that this will become my second home, and at times the only home I can come to. The Kim family will take me in after multiple inpatient admissions, they will welcome me to their dinner table when things get too difficult between me and my parents, and they will treat me like their daughter. They will accept me unconditionally.

I'm the youngest person on the varsity cross country team, and the other girls are hesitant to accept me. My name has been overhyped in local running circles and by my overly proud older sister. The juniors and seniors are welcoming, but the sophomores, too young to find me adorable but too cool for me at the same time, decide that I need a more thorough

Freshman Treatment, which is their form of good-natured hazing. I'm willing, even eager, to endure the Freshman Treatment to become one of the pack, and endure it I do.

"I'll have a scotch on the rocks, hold the scotch," I'm instructed to say after sauntering up to the Olive Garden bar at our first team dinner. The older girls emphasize how important it is to wear my finest gown to our first dinner on the road. I arrive in a sparkly black prom dress, only to realize that everyone else is in the team warm-ups. I'm charged with lugging the team's bags off the bus and always stuck sitting closest to the chaperones. I jump through the necessary hoops, and with Angela vouching for me, I embark on the best three years of my life. I'd never had more in common with any group of girls, and I never have since.

But my best friend, the person I want to sit next to every chance I get, is Angela. We share the exact same sense of humor. She tells me one Friday that her weekend plans are to collect her pee in an empty milk jug, just so she can measure how much she makes. At her behest we fill a bathtub with milk and Corn Pops, because there's no reason not to. She's the kind of odd that borders on weirdo, but she's not, and everybody is drawn to her. When I'm with Angela, it feels like I've found my friend soulmate. Things we do that would raise eyebrows if we did them alone are accepted as two quirky friends going on adventures.

I find comfort in the way she sees food. She thinks calories are bad, but she also does not let them run her life like I do.

She tries to order off the low-calorie menu at restaurants, runs extra when she eats extra, and has a nimble, tiny body that I use as a template for what I could look like one day if I loosened up. Under her influence, I have the occasional ice cream cone and cut a few distance runs short. What doesn't seem fair is that Angela is a garbage disposal. She monitors her calories, but I quickly realize that she is blessed with an insanely high metabolism, or a tapeworm, and she keeps a gymnast's body no matter what. Angela never had a tummy in her baby pictures.

It's not only Angela that helps me slip out of my eating disorder's grip. Initially, running on a team has an extremely positive influence on me. Carb loading is common practice the night before races. In acts of normal teenage defiance, we occasionally play hookie from practice, hiding out behind the equipment shed to play truth or dare games to see who will eat a petunia from a manicured lawn or ring a doorbell and run away. The purpose of running becomes speed and teamwork, and burning calories is a secondary benefit. I gain a few pounds, and for a brief period of time I'm less obsessed with the mirror.

Our assistant coach, Coach Maddox, is a 23-year-old intern who is training for the Olympic Trials. She's so attractive that even after a fateful day at the salon, or more likely SuperCuts, she shows up with a mullet and still catches the eye of everyone she passes. All the boys on the team want to marry her and every girl wants to hate her but can't. Her genuine interest in all of our lives, not just our times on race day, exemplify what a role model should be. If I tell a joke that makes her laugh, I replay it in my head for days. I want her to like me, and the two tools I have at my disposal are humor and speed. I try way too hard in both.

Coach Maddox is the first strong female I idolize, holding her up on a pedestal that she always manages to reach. If she wants me to eat a bagel and banana before a race, she doesn't need to nag me at all. An article from her about proper nutrition for athletes cuts right through my eating hang-ups. Before I know it, I look forward to gatherings at the Olive Garden for pasta dinners before competitions.

I accept a small amount of weight gain as a necessary evil if I want to perform well at meets. I realize my six-pack abs are not worth feeling weak and tired during track workouts and that disappointing times in races are not worth veins in my arms. I don't like the way that my stomach looks when my uniform rides up to reveal that I no longer have abs, but as I get closer to my goals it matters less. Earning Coach Maddox's respect replaces my allegiance to my eating disorder. Coach Maddox is all-knowing, and if her training plan calls for a rest day, I rest. I do whatever she tells me to, convinced that she has the recipe for happiness and success.

My freshman season ends in disappointment. I perform poorly at the state meet and am part of the reason for our Runner Up trophy. I still have the pictures, our eyes swollen from crying as we hold up the consolation prize. The first weekend of the off season, I realize there is no more training plan and Coach Maddox won't be telling me what to do for months. I mourn the loss of structure.

I call Angela. "Do you want to have a crazy weekend?" She's intrigued.

We make plans to erect a gingerbread house. It's November, so a bit early, but our plans are unfolding nicely. Saturday night we assemble a gingerbread house using a kit. It collapses instantly. While I search through my mom's junk drawer for Gorilla Glue to keep it together, Angela starts popping M&Ms into her mouth. I join her, justifying my own indulgence by hers, and between the two of us we devour the whole house.

We both are left with stomach aches, and even though Angela's eating is usually a way to gauge my own, I know we've overindulged. As we lie on the couch, I run my hand up and down my soft stomach, deeply regretting my actions. I look over at Angela and wonder if she too wants to crawl out of her skin.

"Hey Angela, what if tomorrow we had a day where all we did was exercise?" She's surprisingly receptive. "We could just do one thing after another to see how long it takes until we can't do any more. We could be like those ultra-marathon runners."

We pause *Grey's Anatomy*, assuming Meredith and McDreamy will reunite eventually, and move back to the kitchen table to map out our Exercise Marathon.

First, we'll wake up and run ten miles down what we refer to as Spooky Trail because the archway of tree branches seems like perfect scenery for the Headless Horseman. Next, we'll rollerblade, which is not embarrassing if we do it together. We'll go all the way to Hickory Hill and then turn around to make it exactly six miles. Then we'll pack lunch in brown bags as if it's a school day. We can drive to the gym and pick up Diet Cokes from McDonald's on the way. We'll lift weights for two hours, but mostly just as an excuse to sit down. Once we're rested from the weights, we can spend an hour on the elliptical as we watch raunchy music videos with fancy cars, money stacks, and stripper poles. If there's no spin class going on we can ride the spin bikes for 45 minutes, and if there is, we'll do the class. We can finish up with 100 laps in the downstairs pool.

I instantly feel better about the gingerbread house we ate. We're about to have the silliest, most off-the-wall adventure. Angela and Jen. It seems extreme, but it's just us being us.

It was like an anorexic slumber party and we didn't know it. I loved how being with Angela turned what I felt was a shameful secret into a game. It pains me to look back on some of our favorite memories together and realize that I was the friend egging it on.

There are some differences between Angela's mentality and mine, which becomes apparent the next day. We wake up and Angela has had a change of heart.

"Jen, it sounded fun last night but I want to sleep in now. I'm so tired. We can do it another time," she mumbles as she attempts to roll away from the beeps of my alarm.

Our plan is down on paper. Her backing out now is a disaster. It will kill me.

"Angela, it's going to be so fun. Please! Remember how we said we'd play Never Have I Ever on the run? I promise we can go at whatever pace you want, but this is going to be epic."

After several minutes of pleading, I wear her down. She gets dressed and we begin our adventure, one of us more excited than the other. The run and rollerblade are seamless and we're both still intrigued to test how far we can push our bodies. On our way to the gym, Angela wants to stop for a Snickers Marathon bar. We've already packed low-carb tortillas with lettuce and turkey, as specified in our plan. But it makes me happy to see Angela eat more than me, as long as she'll stay with me while we complete our odyssey.

I wonder how her brain works and how she doesn't feel guilty about the extra energy bar. Has she forgotten about the Skittles and icing last night? Has she considered how many miles of running the Snickers Marathon bar will undo? Doesn't she feel like she owes it to the plan to complete it?

This was back when it was all a game. I still didn't realize my bones were deteriorating, that I was pissing them out with every month that went by that I missed my period. But can you miss something you never had? It will be three more years before I'm honest with a doctor, when she'll run the tests and inform me that my hypothalamus and pituitary gland have decided that it's too late. I will never get a period.

In ninth grade I knew my mom was worried that I still hadn't gotten my Woman Pass. So one night after dinner, I called her to my room and told her the big news that I needed her to buy me tampons. She was ecstatic that I'd finally reached this milestone, and for the next year I pretended to menstruate every month. Until Rebecca Mays and her nosy doctor mom ruined it all.

"Jen, can I ask you a question?" Mom asks me after school one day. "Why is there never any blood on the applicators you throw away?"

"Mom, that's so gross. Why would you ask me that?" To be honest, I have no idea what an applicator is and no clue how to insert a tampon.

"Jen, I know it's awkward, but Rebecca's mom said that you will lose bone strength if you don't get your period. She's skeptical you are still getting yours as thin as you are. Rebecca says you throw your lunch away at school. You aren't lying to me, are you?"

"Mom, I swear to God I'm getting my period. I would never even think to lie about that. Dr. Mays is weird."

Still, I know that Mom's suspicious. I have to do something to ease her mind so I can escape her scrutiny. So that evening, I know what must be done. I hate that I have to do it. The idea of cutting myself has always made me nauseous, and I've never understood the girls at school who slit their wrists for an emotional release. But I love running and I love being skinny, and there's a price to pay for both.

I get out of the shower and dry my legs off. I don't want to slice too deep, just enough to draw blood. I need enough to put along the edge of my underwear and on the applicators Mom is apparently examining now. This will erase all doubt. It takes a few tries to get up the nerve. I cringe as the blade sinks into the wrinkled skin over my Achilles tendon. I apply just enough pressure as I move it horizontally. There's a one second delay, and then the blood comes gushing out. I smear the red over as many applicators as I can until there's none left. I milk the wound for every last drop and save the applicators in my lockbox, hoping there are enough to last me six months. I won't have to do this again for at least six months, I tell myself, and I take great comfort in that fact.

A few months later, Angela pauses *Elf* during our standard movie night and tells me she has a confession.

"Jen, I used to drink in middle school." There's gravity in her words.

I'm sheltered by my eating disorder and my parents, and at fourteen, this shocks me. My sister had been vehemently against drinking until she went to college, at which point she turned a drastic 180. I've never been at a party with alcohol and I can't believe that Angela would be involved in something so mischievous. Alcohol ruins lives.

Angela continues. "I wanted to let you know something fun we could do next weekend, but I don't want you to judge me.

My sister bought a handle of vodka and she said we could come over and pregame with her and her roommates before they go out."

I'm hesitant. "I don't know, Angela. If we get caught drinking, I'll be in so much trouble."

It's true. My sister hadn't shattered any glass ceilings for me in that arena. I know my sister would disapprove, but I decide this is a once in a lifetime opportunity. Angela's sister has a strobe light in her dorm room on top of it all!

I have no memory of being at the dorm except for that I keep repeating the same story, something about how my sister doesn't drink but she did once on a cruise. I do know with absolute certainty that I am extremely annoying, and I don't know if the college girls were planning on bringing us to the party, but Angela and I find ourselves back at her house by 9 p.m., banging into her NSYNC and Enrique Iglesias-adorned door as we stumble into her bedroom.

"Vodka, I want more vodka." I'm demanding it, stumbling around her room, checking under her bed and inside her drawers.

"Jen, I don't have any. What are you doing?" She moves toward me in slow motion.

Within two minutes we're jumping around on her bed, squealing about how cute Coach Lance is and how we would totally marry him. Then I say the words that I have known deep in my core since I was twelve years old.

"Angela, I have a secret and it's a really big one. Like, if you tell anybody, if you tell any little person ever, it will ruin my life," I say, trying to separate each word but hearing them smear together against my tongue.

"I promise, pinky promise, one thousand percent forever. It's in the vault," she says, struggling to make the gesture of locking her lips with a key. The vault is where we keep secrets so deep that anyone knowing would destroy our lives, and at this point there are so many secrets in that vault that it's running out of storage.

"I'm anorexic, Angela." I look her in the eye like I'm coming out of the closet, still bouncing as I say it. "I'm fucking anorexic."

I say it assertively, firmly, definitively, and it feels wonderful. I've never said these words out loud to myself, let alone somebody else, and it's freeing to be unapologetically me. I don't want help. I just want her to know who I am.

Angela hugs me hard and begins to cry, tears of happiness. "Jen, so am I."

We're still jumping, hugging each other for balance. I look back at her. "I wanna go down down down."

"I want to go with you. I want to so bad, so bad."

Her bed squeaks under the weight of our confessions, demons we're treating with a levity that will only lead to darkness.

I open my eyes the next morning and the room is swimming. What I'm experiencing is not a hangover. I'm still very drunk, but in my stupor I take note of the bright sun streaming through her window. I smell the sharp odor of vodka, stomach acid, and stir-fry vegetables and I almost get sick again. I am pleased at the unexpected loss of my dinner last night but also disappointed that I ruined my favorite purple Abercrombie shirt. The one I was wearing when Jake asked me out.

I look at my watch. 9:15. I'm a summer camp counselor for a track camp that began over an hour ago. I panic, not because I'm afraid of my boss, who I correctly predict will laugh at me. But because I realize I won't be there when my mom comes to pick me up. I shake Angela awake, switching my strategy to targeted poking when she tries to push me off of her.

"Angela, I need you to drive me to the track now. If I'm not there before my mom, my life is over." Angela rouses and stumbles to her sink.

My amnesia from the night before, a curtain made of vodka, blocks my memory momentarily. Why do I feel like there is something different when I look at her? Then I remember, and realize I've revealed something that will destroy me if it gets out. No vault in the world is secure enough to contain this secret.

"Angela, do you remember what I said last night? That thing about being anorexic? I don't know why I said that. I was just being weird, but I was lying."

She looks at me, confident in her response, and says, "I wasn't."

We don't speak of this night again for two years.

I Don't Fuck With You

It was cathartic breaking up with Jake. He was not a kind boyfriend. He would Eddie Haskell his way through dinners with my parents, a squeaky-voiced class clown who would easily blend in on the cover of *Kids Abercrombie*. We're fourteen and we both look about ten. It's so adorable. The two tiniest people in ninth grade are dating. People love the idea of Jake and Jen.

But Jake has another side, a passive aggressive side. He ditches me at parties to make the more popular girls laugh. "Your boyfriend is straight up hilarious," the cool girls tell me. But I'm starting to not find him so funny.

I always feel half-witted around Jake, my academic prowess a poor surrogate for common sense. Jake takes objective truths and adds his own seasoning, spinning things until the floor and ceiling are indistinguishable.

I'm smarter than him, and it's a constant point of contention. I'm cautious not to rub in my more rigorous course load.

"You got an A on your *Beowulf* essay? Ms. Irving is an easy grader. I don't know why they have her teaching AP. Mr. Sylvester makes Pre-AP seem like AP. If he had been your teacher, there's no way you could have gotten higher than a B," he tells me matter-of-factly.

I'm faster than him, which is an even more sensitive topic.

"Running is all you're good at though. You can't skateboard or play the guitar. I'm learning guitar, did I mention that?"

Even my first kiss, shared with Jake himself, is polluted with the stench of competition. We're standing in my driveway after a game of HORSE, a pollen-covered Spalding basketball tucked under my arm. The prize if I won was a kiss on the cheek. The prize if Jake won was a kiss, with tongues. I threw the game. It's the heat of the day on a Sunday afternoon, and Jake walks closer, his linen Hawaiian shirt grazing my arm, tickling my skin.

"Have you ever made out with somebody?" he asks, never one to mince words.

"No, not yet," I say, hoping this will soon change.

"Are you serious? You've never kissed anybody?"

Suddenly I feel about two inches tall.

"I kissed Chase Wilson on New Year's in sixth grade." I'm slightly defensive. It was true, a peck on the lips right as the ball dropped. I'd asked my mom for permission, of course.

Y2K could have ended the world that night, and I didn't want to freefall into the apocalypse having never kissed a boy.

"Yeah, but were there tongues?" Jake is not impressed.

"Well, no," I concede.

"I can't believe you're in ninth grade and you've never made out with anybody. I've made out with lots of girls. I'm a really good kisser." His tone softens and he leans in. As he sticks his tongue in my mouth and swirls it around, I realize he is the best kisser I've ever experienced. Somehow he sends tingles up and down my spine and my Reef sandals nearly lift straight off my driveway. Then my dad comes out, searching for a power tool that, looking back, was a poorly crafted excuse to prematurely end this magical moment.

Jake and I begin to take advantage of the gap between the dismissal bell and track practice. We always have a few minutes to get changed before Coach Donaldson pulls up in his beat-up pickup, stumbles to the track with his one glass eye, and fumbles through a speech, the after-effects of years of alcoholism coating every word with a fuzzy layer of confusion.

"Girls, go run ten...uh, girls, go run ten miles. Be back in thirty minutes." Math was not a strength for Coach Donaldson.

Today, Jake and I wait in his older sister's punch buggy listening to Eminem's latest hits. He puts his hand on my arm and I think maybe we will make out again. I like kissing him. He was right, he's a really good kisser. Lots of tongue, but he tastes like Sprite and I like that. But he seems alarmed, genuinely concerned by something on my arm. Is there a precancerous mole? A scorpion? What could be so horrifying, able to kill the mood of a 3 p.m. makeout session?

"Oh my God!" he exclaims.

"What? What is it?" I jerk forward in my seat, expecting a snake to slither past me.

His hand is still on my arm and he sinks his fingers into my skin. "Your arm feels like mayonnaise! Why is it so squishy?"

I'm not used to comments about being fat. The callouses I once formed against these remarks as a husky child have softened after three years of recreational anorexia, the door still open for me to slip out if I choose. His words pierce through my layer of mayonnaise and settle somewhere in my bloodstream, reactivating the virus that lay dormant for months.

"What do you mean? No it doesn't." I need this not to be true. I need him to be kidding, to take it back.

"Feel my arm, Jen." He flexes his muscle and a ping pong ball emerges from a bone.

"Feel that. Pinch it. There's no squish on top. Now feel yours. Why is yours so squishy? It's like it's all fat."

Suddenly, in the only way he could have twisted this situation, Jake has made my skinniness into fatness.

"Jake, I'm really skinny. My doctor doesn't even like it. My mom makes me drink Ensure every day when she picks me up."

It's true. What I omit is that I sneak into the fridge at night, dump out the chocolatey sabotage, and refill the opaque bottles with tap water, often not having the luxury of time to properly rinse them out. Consequently, after practice each day I am greeted with cloudy tap water, which I chug with an exaggerated smacking of the lips so Mom will believe I'm on board with my pediatrician's plan.

"Well think about it Jen. We're the same exact weight and I'm a guy."

Jake, I should add, is an anomaly, perhaps the smallest human being possible. We are tied at 89 pounds and whoever hits 90 first will be the unspoken loser. After a long run you can see his heart pulsate in his chest, his xiphoid process and rib cage on full display. I try to play it off, as if his comment, so nonchalantly delivered, has not just wrecked my world.

"I'll just do some extra pushups. It's not because I weigh too much. I've just been focused on running and I haven't been able to do as many pushups." I am once again the sixth grader in the fish-patterned one piece, telling Hannah my summer weight loss has already been scheduled and my love handles were premeditated.

But that night at dinner, I decide maybe I don't need that extra serving of rice, maybe all this carb loading is really the pathway to obesity. Some nights I haven't bothered to throw up my ice cream in the shower. Lazy, I think. I'm getting sloppy and it's starting to show.

I have a very honest look in the full-length mirror after my shower. I flex, lean back, and contort my body like a snake. I can't see my bottom two abs. The tennis ball that used to emerge when I flexed my arm is gone. There's no muscle left. I look like Gumby, nothing like the bodybuilders on the cover of *Men's Fitness*. I pull out the album insert to Usher's *Confessions* album. Six-pack abs. Why don't mine look like that anymore?

My bulging six-pack is gone, replaced by endless pasta and breadsticks with my teammates, tapered workout schedules to peak for races, and a state championship ring that was disappointingly anticlimactic. Coach Maddox knew how to get results, but she didn't tell me I'd have to sacrifice my six-pack.

Jake is not finished reminding me that I am Mayonnaise Girl, and by the end of the month I wonder if I should be a spokesperson for Hellman's. I'm ashamed. I know that if I tell anybody what is happening, if I admit it bothers me, they will know that I have an eating disorder. Every adult in my life is trying to make me gain weight. If I admit Jake's comments hurt me, that he's getting under my skin, it will be a huge red flag.

"I'm sure he's just kidding," I imagine friends saying dismissively. But he's not kidding and it doesn't stop.

Finally, out in the school courtyard at lunch, I snap. "Jake I'm tired of you calling me fat." My voice quavers, unable to conceal my pent-up fury. My face is hot and I know that I'm beet red as my armpits sweat under the noon sun.

"What? I'm just joking around. Being pudgy isn't that big of a deal. It's not like you're straight up fat. Why are you being so sensitive? You're skinny fat." Jake looks bewildered.

"If you say it one more time I'm dumping you, Jake. I mean it." My fists clutch my brown lunch bag as I twist it around and around, the paper tearing between my fingers.

"Fine babe, no more jokes. I didn't realize you were so sensitive." Jake takes me under his arm and kisses me, apologizing that we've had our first tiff.

Jake lasts about two days, but my mayonnaisy appearance is too hard for him to resist commenting on. It was cathartic to break up with him, satisfying to hear his tears on the other end of the line, the sniffles and pleas that he won't do it again. But I carry his comments with me. I've let myself down. I've chosen speed over aesthetics. Luckily, the season ends and I decide to get back in the gym, to be more diligent with my crunches and pushups, and to recapture the skinny-buff look I'd earned in seventh grade.

I find motivation in my World Cultures teacher, Ms. Parks. I doodle along the border of my paper as she drones on about triangular trade and Mesopotamia. She's passionate and almost slams the chalk into the board as she writes. But all I can focus on is the flap of skin that used to be a tricep swinging back and forth, gaining enough momentum to continue its jiggle long after she has finished writing her bullet point. I imagine myself digging my fingers into this flap, clinging to it like a monkey, and swinging back and forth. I'm in a loincloth like Tarzan and her flappy arm is a vine I use to propel myself though the understory of the jungle. The thought becomes intrusive, the ninth grade version of Ms. Moon's gnats, and I relish the days she wears her cardigan sweater so I can focus.

Before long I drop all the extra weight that I put on during cross country season, and I'm now confident, with arms that don't look like a condiment. I had to be disciplined and miss a few team gatherings, but you can't put a price on liking what you see in the mirror.

What I didn't realize was that I'd fallen for the Birds of a Feather Principle. If there is a way for anorexics to find each other, fan each other's flames, and perpetuate each other's neuroses, they will find it. Cross country teams are a great place to start.

I see Jake at a craft festival many years later. He's now a grown hipster. He comes over and gives me a side hug, and we briefly catch up. Neither of us is married, no children to feign interest in to carry the small talk. The cute little prep in the Hollister polo, blonde surfer haircut, and Puka shell necklace has been replaced by a grungy man, hair past his shoulders and an aroma indicating he might use natural deodorant. He leads guided tours around Alaska, but I don't remember the details because all I can focus on is the answer to my mayonnaise arms written all over his face, the glaring explanation for his cruel jokes so many years ago.

Jake Kelly is anorexic, a blatant eating disorder hidden behind his gender. Neither of our adorable weights had been what our bodies wanted, and in the strange way tortured souls attract each other, I somehow managed to find the one boy at my high school who weighed less than me and considered me fat. His knobby elbows and knees, the joints thicker in diameter than his actual arms and legs, and the long sunken face I've seen in the mirror so many times over the years, tell me everything I wish I'd known when I was fourteen. He looks more like a haggard 45-year-old than the 30-year-old he should be. At this moment, I finally understand that his comments were never about me. I'd let his eating disorder voice intertwine with mine, lure it out of hibernation, and ignite the ember that had never been properly snuffed out; and for the next sixteen years my brain will be engulfed in flames.

Truth Hurts

Senior year there's an unspoken understanding that childhood is waning, soon to be replaced with deployments, dorm rooms, minimum wage jobs, and unplanned babies. A camaraderie forms between each graduating class, facilitated by proms, senior nights, and graduation rehearsals. Unfortunately, when all of my friends are seniors, I am still a junior and am excluded from these bonding moments. The graduation of the class of 2006 is the end of my social life.

I'm relieved when Angela decides to stay in town for college. She assures me we will still be best friends. I can visit her in her dorm room any time. We are inseparable, and college will not change that.

But her stories begin to revolve around her new roommate, who has a fake ID and knows all the bouncers downtown. Angela's Facebook wall is now filled with pictures of midtown bars, Saturday tailgates, and dorm room air hockey tournaments. My texts linger for days, and when she finally responds, it's usually to emphasize how busy she is with classes, swamped and overwhelmed with a heavy pre-med course load. But that's not what I see on Facebook.

Adding to my hurt is that her random roommate, Vanessa, is the star of Angela's stories. Vanessa did the funniest thing at the Kappa Theta kegger. Vanessa wears the coolest custom Nikes. Vanessa throws the wildest parties. I wonder how Angela has forgotten our original verdict on Vanessa, that she's a compulsive liar and a social climber.

"He's like a brother to me," Vanessa would say smugly about various football players, exaggerating their bond just because they were lab partners in Chemistry or sat next to each other in Geology. Vanessa is also tainted. She had a serious bout with anorexia the previous year and had to take medical leave from college. So even though she is a freshman, she should be a sophomore. She's gained the weight back, but she's proven that she has that sneaky, manipulative vanity that anorexia reveals.

To my pleasant surprise, several months into the fall semester Angela asks me if I want to go for a run, an eight-miler. She pulls up in her silver Acura, Britney Spears' bubbly voice booming through her speakers. One of the things I love most about Angela is that she isn't afraid to hold on to her childhood and sees nothing wrong with returning from a frat party or Microbiology lecture to a bed filled with stuffed animals.

We don't go inside, and after a short greeting we start our trek. We struggle for content to fill the miles, and the laughs that usually come so freely are truncated, meeting early demises as we search for common ground. Then she reveals to me what will change my entire life and cast a sober lens on our drunken night more than two years ago.

"Jen, I need to tell you something. I'm seeing a therapist."

This isn't that big of a deal to me. I'm still on Prozac to prevent an OCD relapse and remember vividly my time with Dr. Krause, the munchkin exterminator. But before I have a chance to promise her that she's not alone, and that this doesn't make her weak or crazy, she continues.

"I'm anorexic. My parents think it's depression but it's not. Vanessa and I went on a diet together and it got out of control."

I hate her words. I want her to swallow them, take them back.

"I don't think you're anorexic, Angela. I mean, we eat together," I say, trying to sound casual. I'm in disbelief that she's saying these words under a sunny sky, uninfluenced by the truth serum of vodka bearing the same name. Therapy makes it real. Until there's an official diagnosis it's just a secret between friends, a casual dalliance with weight manipulation.

"Jen, I am. I've been making myself throw up. Vanessa taught me how to purge when I overeat. I kept cheating on

our diet and it was making me miserable, so she taught me."
She's panting now, the sound of our feet slapping across the
wooden bridge over Pelican Creek.

I can't argue with that. Purging is an extreme behavior, and
a stupid one.

"I'm sorry." I will the insincere words past my lips. She's
letting an outsider in, whoever this therapist is.

"Jen, you're anorexic too, and it's really bad. Since I started
talking to my therapist, her name is Rachel, I've realized how
messed up we both are."

I intentionally increase my pace and listen to her breathing
become labored, her words trailing off out of necessity. "I'm
definitely not anorexic, Angela."

We change the subject to her boyfriend's new car or
something I don't care about, banal words littering the
concrete as we leave them in our wake. What bothers me is
that Angela is joining my parents' team. We used to play games
with exercise and counting calories was one of our quirks, no
different than buying Moon Boots to bounce around the
house in. I hate her for being so stupid, for allowing a therapist
to put a diagnosis on what no outsider could comprehend.

Later that night I stand in the shower and turn the knob all
the way to the red **H**. I want to feel my skin burn as I rinse
Angela's weakness off of me, washing her words away. I let
the water scald my skin as I stare at the spigot and wonder if
she's right, knowing in my core, in the place within me that the
water can't cleanse, that she is.

Confessions

By spring of my junior year, my eating disorder, once in remission, is back with a vengeance.

"Honey, you sure are spending a lot of time getting ready for Panther Prowl," Mom would say, looking slightly concerned that I may be burning the candle at both ends. Panther Prowl is a pep rally for our school's mediocre football team, full of skits that make *Saturday Night Live* look hilarious. I hate being in student council and I know I was a legacy pick, only allowed into the inner political circle of my high school because my sister was treasurer of the class of 2004.

Panther Prowl is really my excuse to drive around listening to Lil Jon & the East Side Boyz and sit outside of Subway leisurely devouring Veggie Delite salad with mustard and Sweet'n Low. I ponder the irony. I'm losing weight and firming up, but my whole life revolves around eating.

After the vegetables I go to the gym, determined to never let my arms be mistaken for a mushy condiment again. My favorite exercise is tricep pushdowns, where I can feel the muscle pop out as I straighten my arms, making my softness hard, erasing the weakness of femininity from my body. I look at the meatheads who carry around duffle bags filled with HGH and TRT. If only I could be like one of those veiny men with no neck, lamenting over how much food I have to eat as my biceps bulge, not an ounce of fat to cover them. I can't decide if I'm attracted to them, want to look like them, or both.

When it's time to return for track season, I'm faster than ever. I'm a contender to compete individually in the state championships for the 3200. But my diet gets in the way. I hyperventilate during track workouts and wheeze during races, wildly inconsistent from one meet to the next. I develop a hairline crack in my foot and have to sit out the middle of the season. This leads me to overcompensate with swim workouts and develop more fear around food now that I'm unable to run. When I return, passing out becomes a regular occurrence, sometimes during track workouts but several times at actual meets. Luckily, my body usually waits until the finish line, but the **DNF** (did not finish) abbreviation is printed in the local paper beside my name more than once. The passion is gone for me. Running is now a means to burn calories and earn food.

If you break 11:16 you can have Sun Chips and a 6-inch turkey sub at Subway tonight. If you don't, you'll need to get a Veggie Delite salad with salt and mustard.

These are the thoughts that circle around in my head as I hear the last lap bell for the 3200 and try not to let my pace drop. This is not the mentality of a winner. The voice is not mean or overtly abusive. This is business. I have chosen a particular lifestyle, and to fulfill the requirements of said lifestyle there are actions I must take. I end the season injured, skipping the rest days on my training plan until the stress fracture in my foot returns.

Parents and teachers whisper about me, their words not yet evaporated when I enter a room. Other parents harass my mother, questioning whether she feeds me. It's not her fault. My pediatrician will later tell me I should join the CIA or become a spy, because in lieu of forming meaningful high school memories, I spend my days plotting every possible scenario that could sabotage my weight loss and preemptively countering them one by one.

Step 1: Never let anybody see my weight. I keep a lockbox in my trunk that holds ankle weights, sodium-filled bouillon cubes, and salt packets, tools to help me bloat myself and cheat the scale when I'm dragged to my pediatrician.

Step 2: Save eating for situations that matter. Eating in front of schoolmates isn't nearly as important as eating in front of my family. People at school aren't going to cancel my gym membership or send me off to treatment. Thanksgiving with the entire extended family is crucially important. My appearance is a source of humiliation for my mom, a condemnation of her parenting skills. So for two weeks prior to family events, I bank calories. I shave off 200 a day for a week until I have 1400 spare calories to splurge on. Nobody will be concerned if my plate is piled high and I'm laughing heartily, defending my Yahtzee title.

Step 3: Counteract all weight gain efforts. Dr. Cartman recommends whole milk at dinner, an easy way to squeeze in extra calories. So after my parents are asleep, I replace half the milk in the gallon with water. It's a delicate balance. If I dilute it too much, it will be apparent I've tampered with it. When my mom insists that she pack my lunch again, filling it with high calorie nuts and cheeses, I buy diet foods to keep in my locker.

Step 4: Over-exercise. I never snuck out to go to parties in high school. I did, however, fabricate study sessions and movie nights to slip off to the gym and run on the treadmill.

Step 5: Purge, but come up with a different name for it so I don't have to acknowledge it. Purging is dangerous. Only really sick, messed up girls purge. I "spit up." It's harmless, and I don't stick my fingers down my throat. I can only do it with ice cream, and I prefer to regurgitate in the shower where the evidence falls down the drain. I end up eating a lot of ice cream and taking a lot of showers. I like ice cream, I like being clean, and it's not like I'm actually purging solid food.

The problem with these steps, besides the fact that I'm wasting memorable years on meaningless games, is that the harder my parents try to help me, the more weight I lose. Trying to put on a show for Thanksgiving means starving myself in advance. Knowing that I will come home to a meal covered in butter means no breakfast or lunch. The more weight I lose, the more my parents try new techniques to help me. And round and round we go.

My mom often looks at me and contorts her face into an expression that makes sure I know that she wants to cry. "What have I done to be such a terrible mother? You're looking like this to embarrass me. Do you know what it's like to go to an awards ceremony and have all the other parents ask me what I feed you? You're doing this to spite me, to get payback, to be passive aggressive."

It all comes to a head a week before Christmas. After my sister leaves for college there is no distraction from me, and the only thing noteworthy about me at this point is my weight. I detect tension when I get home from school and hear muffled whispers in my parents' bedroom. I press my ear against the door.

"Tom, something is wrong. Don't try to smooth it over like you always do. You just don't want to deal with the fallout. You'd rather watch your daughter waste away than rock the boat. She looks like shit and nothing we try works."

"Debbie, I never said nothing was wrong. I just said maybe if we back away and let her figure it out on her own, things will get better. She's got a good group of friends and she's trying. She's just stubborn. But maybe it is at the point where we need to intervene."

"Even Natalie said it's gotten out of hand. Do you know what she ate for a snack when she visited her at the dorms? Salty lettuce. Natalie bought her a pint of Ben and Jerry's and she said she wanted salty lettuce instead. Somebody who really wants to gain weight doesn't do that, Tom."

The salty lettuce was a mistake. I thought I could let my guard down for a weekend away from my parents. I flinch at my stupidity.

My mom continues. "I'm going to take her to get checked for cancer over Christmas break. This is either anorexia or cancer. We are getting to the bottom of this. I'm not waiting around anymore, Tom."

I freeze. The color drains from my cheeks and a clammy chill fills my chest. I'm tired of them asking questions, tired of feeling like I've swallowed thumb tacks when I go to the doctor, tired of bloating myself with bouillon cubes to trick the scale, tired of the deceit.

I open the door. I don't care if they know I was eavesdropping. I want to come clean.

"I'm anorexic," I say, no buffer, no introduction. "I'm fucking anorexic." It's the second time I've said these words out loud and the first time I've said them sober.

Jen II emerges for the first time. This is her birth place. To this day, whenever my anorexia is exposed or challenged, a defiant, ornery alter ego emerges, dropping f-bombs even in places they don't fit very well. I've come to realize Jen II won't go away until every bit of my anorexia is gone, because they are one in the same.

I've tried to be agreeable for the past four years, hiding how furious the Ensures make me, pretending to relish the buttered dinners when I want to smash the plate against the wall, suppressing the urge to take the birthday pancakes and shove them up my mom's ass.

"Okay, honey, it's okay. Everything is okay. We can solve this." My dad, always the rational scientist, goes into fix-it mode. "If you eat a third of a Snickers bar every two hours-"

I roar, explode, erupt with four years of pent-up aggression. "I don't want a fucking Snickers bar. I just told you I'm anorexic. No, no, no, no. Fuck Snickers. Fuck it." I twitch, tug at my skin, and scratch at my neck as I writhe in the agony of the truth.

My mom fumes and directs her pain at my dad. "I told you, Tom. I've told you for four years and now look what happened. You told me everything was okay and I was just being paranoid, a helicopter mom. Look at her. This is your fault. I will never forgive you."

Since the shit has already hit the fan, I decide there's no harm in adding to the splatter. I want to be open and I want to get better. I'm a kid and I assume there's some adult who will have the answers. It will be a tough struggle, but this monkey will be off my back. There's a solution an adult will have, some deep-seated piece of me I'm just not seeing. My brain is locked and I just need someone to help me crack the code.

"Mom, Dad, I'm not really 95 pounds." I tell them about the lockbox. My dad follows me to my car where I reveal my container of deceit. I line up the combination numbers and give him my ankle weights, my bouillon cubes, and the salt packets. I lift the trunk liner that houses my spare tire and surrender my digital scale, the one that tells me when I can stop chugging as I sit outside of my pediatrician's office.

I no longer have anything to lose. My skeletons are out of the closet, and as I hand over my exceedingly heavy contraband, I fittingly feel like a great weight has been lifted.

I'm Different

I'm terrified to begin therapy for an eating disorder. The munchkins were clearly fake, but looking better when I'm thin is very much real. Angela tells me that Rachel has a good body and will not try to make me fat. She promises me Rachel is cool, not pushy like Dr. Cartman and Rebecca Mays's mom.

I've never known a Rachel and can't imagine who this person is doling out weight gain advice but who seems to be liked nonetheless. I form a mental picture of her; blonde hair, horn-rimmed glasses, feet propped up on a chair as she dispenses wisdom about my inner child. Maybe a cigar hanging out of the side of her mouth.

As I sit between my parents in her surprisingly small lobby, I try to decide how much to reveal. When she walks out, she's nothing like I pictured. She doesn't look old enough to have wisdom. She's older than Coach Maddox, but not like the therapists in my Lifetime movies that twirl their pencils around as they help their patients realize that their husbands are trying to kill them. She looks more like an older sister, possibly the prettiest person I've ever seen. I'm relieved that she's not overweight. I was expecting somebody rotund, somebody who wanted me to be fat like them, but she is slender. I look at her stomach and it's definitely not distended. I wonder if she has a six-pack. She must.

Here I am, a head full of mixed-up puzzle pieces. I wonder where she'll start. How will she assemble all the pieces, leaving me with a brain that looks like the picture on the box? I imagine the climax of a movie where the therapist finally discovers the key that fits and unlocks just the right cortex, freeing the patient from their agony as the Northern Lights illuminate the sky.

I instantly like her when I see her suppress a chuckle as my mom melodramatically tells her about the ankle weights and lockbox. She doesn't think I'm a tragic character in an after school special. Not yet. I wonder if she's going to make me gain weight. She seems relatable enough to let that slide.

I want help. I don't want to be anorexic. It's destroyed my life and it's tearing my parents up. I can't focus at school and I'm always freezing cold. I want a family one day, I want to be able to go out to restaurants, and I want a normal life. But I also want to be 85 pounds of pure muscle. I have never been able to reconcile these two desires, but I'm hoping she will help me. I view her as the Coach Maddox of my brain, and I'm eager to learn what her plan will be for my recovery.

Looking back, I think my true desire was to not WANT to weigh 85 pounds any more. I wanted to gain weight and love myself anyways, and be comfortable in a bigger body. What I did not realize was that to recover, I'd have to keep going even on the days I hated what I see in the mirror. Body positivity is a misnomer, much more accurately described as body acceptance. Nobody likes their body all the time, especially not someone prone to the perfectionism and self-hate of anorexia.

Recovery is a sacrifice. A recovering alcoholic will never feel the tantalizing haze of drunkenness again, and that is a loss that he will mourn. An anorexic who truly wants recovery must give up the gratifying sensation of looking in the mirror and seeing bones, sinews and veins, and to her, that too is a meaningful loss. Whatever void anorexia once filled will ache with emptiness, and the only way to recover is to embrace the discomfort and trust that something better lies on the other side.

Rachel asks me to make a list of everything I've lost from my eating disorder. I title it **The Cost of My Eating Disorder**. I thought it was long at the time.

1. **I'm hungry all the time.**
2. **I don't have a period.**
3. **My parents and I are always fighting.**
4. **I can't have boyfriends because I can't eat with them.**
5. **I'm always cold.**

Rachel tells me to view anorexia as an external force so that I don't identify with it. It's not on my side, and I need to stop viewing it as a friend. "It's hard to view something that has felt like a friend as an enemy. But an eating disorder is like a bully who doesn't want you to have any other friends. It wants you all to itself and it's brainwashed you into thinking it's a friend. That voice is not yours."

I give the expected response, that I hate my eating disorder and I want to change. And I truly think I mean it. But as I leave her office, I catch myself comforting my eating disorder. *It's okay. I'm never going to let you get fat. Never again.*

My trust in Rachel helps me make progress in spite of my entrenched thinking patterns. She helps me realize the thoughts that come so naturally to me are ruining my relationships. She doesn't force any dogma on me or stereotypically blame my mother, and this helps me open up. She's the first person I've told about my rituals since Dr. Krause, and she helps me discover that many of my compulsions are now designed to "earn my food." I have to run a certain number of miles so that I'll let myself eat dinner. I have to weigh all of my food on a kitchen scale so that I won't panic mid-bite and throw it all away. The eating disorder is not my friend, and instead of helping me overcome my OCD, it has made all of my compulsions worse by tying them to food.

I can't listen to my body signals yet to tell me how much to eat because I'm too underweight. To have any semblance of a real life I have to gain weight. I want to jump ahead, dive right into the fun parts of recovery and skip the weight gain. Why can't recovery be à la carte?

I gain about five pounds, only because I like Rachel so much. I trust her, and she herself appears to take pride in her appearance, though she's extremely tall and probably has much more leeway with her calories. She reinforces the foreign concept that there are many things better than being thin, like having a social life and enjoying my first year of college. I've never considered that counting calories and losing weight is a colossal waste of time, not a glamorous pursuit of perfection, and suddenly any sense of superiority for my discipline is replaced with embarrassment that these games are my focus.

We set a goal weight of 100 pounds. I get to 90 and I don't feel any better. I still can't think about anything but food, yet I'm still terrified to eat it. The gaping hole, the void inside of me, is worse than ever. The OCD that my restriction had been masking reemerges. Did I accidentally eat two sandwiches today at lunch? I start digging through the trash, hoarding wrappers to line them up and check them over and over again like model dogs being shielded from a house fire. I commit to a meal plan that is higher in calories, but this too becomes a compulsion. I used to eat as little as possible, and now that I am trying to eat more, I realize I have no idea how to serve a normal plate.

I throw temper tantrums at the dinner table, mainly directing my wrath at my mom because she is the one cooking. Rachel mediates and tells my parents that this is quite a normal part of the process and why family therapy is so important. Things usually get worse before they get better.

Rachel requires me to see a dietician so that I am being medically monitored throughout the process. She refers me to Sharon Sortino, an advocate of intuitive eating. Intuitive eating is based around the set point theory. The human body is designed to settle around a particular weight range predetermined by genetics. When it's above this range appetite will naturally decrease, and when it's below this range it will increase. Sharon has recovered from an eating disorder in her own life and wants to help others get out of the endless hole of diets and restriction.

As I sit in the waiting room, I hear the trickle of a fountain flowing over the stone carving of a cherub. I wonder if Sharon thinks he is the appropriate weight. His stomach is not flat, and if he weren't carved in stone, I'm sure it would be soft. Within a month, I will hate this cherub as he seduces my overfilled bladder to release.

Because I fully understand intuitive eating, I'm shocked when Sharon gives me a strict, detailed meal plan. My day will revolve around hitting exact numbers of starches, fats, and proteins. It seems like another form of calorie counting, but the target numbers are all much too high for my comfort.

Sharon is not overweight, but I decide I could never accept being in her body. It casts an immediate cloud of suspicion over her advice. She believes, like Rachel, that I am below my set point, and until I reach an appropriate weight I cannot eat intuitively. Like Rachel, she estimates that once I get to 100 pounds I'll be able to start learning appetite cues. When Rachel says it, it doesn't sound as absurd. But Sharon's words drip of ulterior motive. She just wants to make me fat.

"Jen, I've seen people drop out of school after making straight As their entire lives."

I think about my report card, how I've just been nominated valedictorian of my high school, and how my acceptance letter to Brighton University is only a formality. I think about my name in the *Sanford Sun* every weekend for running, how a spot on the Brighton track team is as good as mine. This woman doesn't know that I'm different.

"I've sat across from women who have spent a decade wrestling with the same two pounds."

This is a scare tactic. This will never be me.

I decide I can master intuitive eating while I'm still underweight if I try hard enough, as if it's a test I can cram for. I start tinkering around behind the scenes to create my own recovery plan. There has to be a faster, easier way. Maybe I'm not willing to gain a pound this week, but I'm journaling a lot more. If everyone would just stop dwelling on my weight, I could work on what matters most, which is building a normal life.

So I begin to chug. The days prior to and the hours immediately before being weighed by Sharon were painful, and in hindsight I'm lucky I didn't dilute my electrolytes enough to die. My full bladder, combined with the trickling fountain in the waiting room, were more than I could handle most weeks, and I rarely made it back to my car before peeing behind the manicured shrub in the parking lot. If I had used her bathroom, it would have been obvious I was chugging because I would pee for at least two solid minutes.

I never thought that I was cheating myself. I was the terminally ill cancer patient convinced I could design a better treatment plan than my oncologist. I substituted essential oils for chemotherapy and deluded myself, convinced that I was doing the work. Rachel was the only person on my treatment team I trusted. She knew my fears and vulnerabilities, saw me cry, and validated my feelings. Later I will wonder why she stops trusting me, why she resents me. I was fucking around. I didn't think I was. At the time I thought Sharon was insane and I was doing what was necessary to get around her.

The third component to my treatment is family therapy with Dr. Gerrard. Dr. Gerrard resembles Jack Nicholson, with a gravelly voice and goatee to match. His island T-shirt and flip flops match his relaxed demeanor as he barrels toward retirement. My sister joins us too, and it's oddly reminiscent of all those years ago leaving the Sweetwater Mall after trying on dresses. She's trapped in a minivan of mental illness, but this time it's $85 an hour.

Our first session, Dr. Gerrard illuminates the dysfunctional family dynamic as it pertains to me. My entire family now must walk on eggshells to avoid triggering me. I have more power, he argues, than most normal sixteen-year-olds could ever hope for. Boss Jen, he dubs me, and he leans over to shake my hand for dramatic effect. "It's good to meet you, Boss Jen."

I hate him for shoving the truth in my face. Suddenly I would prefer to be seen as the vulnerable victim of anorexia, a damsel in distress. But he points out that I am in an abusive, but nonetheless consensual, relationship with my eating disorder. My illness impacts my entire family. As we leave, I tell my dad I never want to go back. But my dad reminds me that we have to do the hard work that nobody wants to do in order for me to get better.

Our second session shines the spotlight on my mom and goes decidedly differently. Dr. Gerrard's analysis is that my mom has chosen me to be the sick daughter, and having a breakable child helps her justify her decision to stay at home and never finish school. By blaming herself for my issues, she can share in the tragedy and seek comfort from my dad. She uses extended periods of moping as a power play to discourage dissent from other members of the family, and she is more concerned with blaming my dad for my eating disorder than helping me recover.

Like Dr. Starkist, Dr. Gerrard does not know the Debbie Rules. Mom contorts her face into the soulful eyes, the "I-can't-cry-on-command-but-if-I-could-I-would" face.

"You're blaming me for her eating disorder. It's all my fault. I should just leave the family and move away. It would be better for everyone. I've been a terrible mother and now Jen is going to die."

Dr. Gerrard, though I don't remember his precise words, insinuates that this is manipulative behavior. Mom walks out of the session early, presumably to pack her things so she can sleep in the spare room for several weeks. Later that evening, Dad informs me that we will not be continuing family therapy. "We don't need to dredge up every little thing that's ever happened."

This is my treatment plan for the rest of high school. Rachel helps me navigate special events. I go to prom and grad night at Adventure Island. I follow my meal plan for the most part. I keep a detailed journal to process difficult emotions, usually related to my home life. And I actually gain some weight. My primitive ideas about recovery transform, and I decide that instead of being 85 pounds but having no eating disorder behaviors, a worthier goal is to look at why I want to be thin so badly. I want the eating disorder voice gone, and with Rachel's support, I begin to truly view it as the enemy.

"Jen, I want you to have fun in college. There's so much more to life than this eating disorder. It's a waste of your time and you can get better from it, but you have to actually gain weight. You can't recover without gaining weight, and sometimes that is going to mean feeling totally out of control. I've worked with people who eat entire boxes of cereal when they are in the early stages of refeeding. It's a normal response to starvation, and you have to accept that it's part of everyone's recovery journey."

If I had a time machine, I would go back to before I learned to purge, before my bone density was that of an 80-year-old's, before I'd missed out on what should have been the best years of my life. I would actually comprehend her words. Recovery is not only about gaining weight, but accepting the chaos. When Rachel comforts me after a few incidents of eating lunch an hour too early, I do not actually hear what she is saying. I still believe I have a stronger will than any other person she has worked with and that I can defy the laws of physiology.

If Rachel had a time machine, she would probably not defend me. My parents wanted to send me away to an inpatient hospital for the remainder of my senior year. Rachel convinced them to give me a chance. I think this regret, on her part, is why she is so hard on me to this day.

By spring of my senior year, my parents give up on family dinners. Too many of them end with me accusing my mom of adding extra oil or butter to the food as a ploy to make me fat. For the first twelve years of my life, our family ate a very low-fat, high-vegetable diet, and most dishes came out of a Weight Watchers cookbook. When I became underweight, my mom added different things to my meal, but because I was cheating, either feeding it to Buddy under the table or stuffing it in my napkin, it didn't bother me. Once I enter treatment, my goal, and the expectation, is that I eat what my mom cooks, and this leads to many explosive fights.

My mom joins me for one of my dietician sessions. Sharon Sortino also does not know the Debbie Rules and questions my mom's choice to continue serving salad as a main dish for dinner.

"We put lots of things in the salad. Chicken, nuts, dressing... it's a well-balanced meal," my mom tells her.

Sharon believes that in the refeeding stage, salad as a main dish sends mixed signals. My mom leaves the session early after telling Sharon through sobs, "So I did this? My salads are what made her sick? I give up. I can't do anything right."

I still feel conflicted about who was right, Sharon or my mom. I was sitting between two extremes. My mom was doing her best to navigate the conflicting health advice of the early 2000s and Sharon was putting her own experiences with weight bias onto my mom when I'm not sure it applied. But something Sharon said must have stuck, because my mom starts trying unfamiliar recipes made with real butter and cream. The same woman who threw away my Halloween candy as a kid, or gossiped if she saw another mother with donuts in her grocery cart, now pretends as if she never emphasized health or nagged me about my weight.

She makes spaghetti one night, which I know to expect. It's 330 calories a plate according to the Weight Watchers cookbook, and though it's a more challenging meal for me, I feel prepared. The winter chill is finally over, and we decide to eat out on the patio. It almost feels like how it used to before Natalie moved out, and before I had an eating disorder.

I struggle with knowing how much pasta to serve. I'm allowed to use a food scale to pack my lunch, but at dinner my parents help me serve myself enough food. When I try to trust my own eyes, I consistently underestimate how much I should take. When I dip the ladle into the sauce, I see an unwelcome addition to the mix. My mom has added garbanzo beans as if it's no big deal. She may as well have laced the meal with shards of glass. I have no idea how to serve my plate any more. The calorie count in the cookbook is now totally useless. Maybe a few months ago I would have taken a tiny portion and used this as an excuse to restrict, but tonight I'm trying to eat a full meal and I have no idea how to do it.

I lash out at my mom. "Are there beans in here?"

"Yes, I thought it would be a nice addition." She's cheerful, probably looking forward to eating outside and enjoying the warmer weather.

"But there were no beans before." Jen II is becoming a fully formed human being at this phase of my treatment. I'm angry I have an eating disorder, angry I'm in treatment for it, angry my family won't participate in family therapy, angry I can't stay 85 pounds. All of my fury is channeled into the beans. I dump the sauce back in the serving pan. I re-serve my plate, suddenly deciding to face my fear head on. Then I take a bite, spit it back out, and begin a tirade. I'm hungry but I'm scared of my dinner; I'm hopeless, cornered, and out of solutions. My breaths turn to wheezes as I look at a table covered in food and realize that I'll starve tonight.

"Fuck this spaghetti. I can't fucking do this, fuck man. What do I eat? I can't eat. I'm so hungry. I can't eat this fucking food." I've taken it upon myself to revalidate the Fuck Pass I'd tried to use back when I was five.

I get up from the table and pace into the house. I'm red with rage, Mom is sobbing, and Dad futilely attempts to calm us both down. Mom locks herself in her bedroom and then pokes her head into the foyer.

"Jen, I'm never cooking for you again. You can feed yourself. I'm not doing it anymore. Get the fuck out."

This would have been really helpful to process in family therapy.

I'm relieved. This is the kindest thing she has said to me in months, the words I've been longing to hear. Permission to not be monitored at dinner. The last months of high school, I spend my nights eating dinner in the Subway parking lot behind an industrial dumpster listening to angry talk radio. I don't care about the politics, or even agree with what the pundits say. But as I stare down at my plastic bowl of chopped vegetables, I need a voice that matches the one that screams at me every minute of every day. I'm happy that I'm now free to dine alone, but something feels unnatural about eating behind a dumpster, even when you have an eating disorder.

I hold on to the hope that moving out of my parents' house into my own place for college will change things. I wish I could say that's because I want to recover, but subconsciously I want the freedom to waste away. I still believe deep down in my core that there is glamour in starvation and I'll find it if I starve myself enough.

Lose Yourself

I'm so sorry, God. I've taken my life for granted. If you let me come out of this, if you don't let the wild boars gore my insides and root through my body, using my organs as an afternoon snack, if you give me this one more chance, I promise you I'll go to church tomorrow. I promise you I'll call Rebecca Mays even though I hated her in high school. I don't want to die with bad blood between us. It doesn't matter that she told her mom I was anorexic, doesn't matter she snitched and made me cut my Achilles. I'm going to call her if you let me out of this tree. I'm going to call her and ask her to lunch. I'm going to go over to my parents' house and make it right, tell them I'm sorry we couldn't get along in high school. Tell them I'm sorry for all the trouble I caused.

It's 8 p.m. and I'm lost in San Marco State Park. I replay the events that got me here.

It all started in the wee hours of the morning, around 1 a.m. I ransacked my roommate's pantry again. A box of Pop-Tarts, eight Special K bars, and a jar of peanut butter. All gone. All I wanted for my whole life was to live on my own and restrict, no parents to monitor my behavior. Three months later and I've gained six out-of-control, sloppy pounds. I'm 99 disgusting pounds of Pop-Tarts.

If I have to go to Walmart one more night to replace all of Alicia's food, I'll scream. What's wrong with me? I have no willpower.

After my first binge so many weeks ago, I emailed Rachel, bewildered at the beast that had taken over my body for ten minutes and plowed through an entire box of NutriGrain bars. If only these episodes were still so minor.

Jen, this is the body's way of getting you to a healthy weight. Let yourself get to a normal weight and it will stop. You aren't a binge eater. You've been starved since you were twelve. Show yourself some kindness for giving in to normal hunger signals.

Her words did not help. Rachel is one of my favorite humans but her reply was gobbledygook, useless drivel. I have blown a fuse. There's a synapse in my brain that is misfiring. I'm broken.

Eight years of anorexia and I've lost my touch. I've tried everything. Online support groups. Duct taping my unsuspecting roommate's cabinets shut when she goes out of town. Punishing myself with extra workouts to pay for the episodes of depravity.

Nothing worked. My last resort was the cockroaches. Nothing turns my stomach and ruins a meal like a cockroach scuttling along the baseboards, tainting the air. I used this to my advantage. I downloaded fourteen pictures of the largest, crunchiest cockroaches on the internet and hung them on the wall above my desk. I never imagined I'd overeat gazing at a gallery of cockroaches, disheveled wings, spiny legs, and twitchy antennae waiting to come to life and scurry across my food. The pictures alone made me gag.

But alas, just like any other night, Alicia went to bed and I tiptoed into the kitchen, pulled a box of brown sugar cinnamon Pop-Tarts out of her cabinet, and devoured all eight pastries in a frenzy. I didn't even have the decency to toast them or get a plate. I tried not to make eye contact with the German cockroach next to my high school diploma as I forced large, dry globs down my throat. I tried to tell my central nervous system that they were just pictures, that I didn't need to reflexively jump out of my chair and squeal or close my eyes and compose myself before swatting them down.

No, joined by an audience of fourteen cockroaches, I earned myself a day of fasting. I've tried to puke. I've jammed perfume-coated fingers down my throat until I feel I might suffocate. I've twisted and gagged, jumped up and down, humped the air on all fours, and the only thing I've ever been able to purge is ice cream. But that skill is not helping me anymore. It's no match for Alicia's pantry of sin.

I knew my day was ruined. I knew I'd cave to peer pressure later. Not the toxic kind, but the kind that dares to tear me away from my eating disorder for another night of fun. After a few pleadings from Michelle, I knew I'd be convinced to chug down vodka shots, guzzle beer, and dance with boys who mention brunch the next day. I knew I'd be weak and take the extra shot, stand on my head, and freestyle rap to a crowd of strangers.

The roaches witnessed me eat all of my allotted food for two days, but I made a deal with myself that if I exercised for long enough, I could drink unlimited vodka with my friends that night. I drove to Walmart to replace what I took. I planned to slip the boxes back in Alicia's pantry so she'd be none the wiser. As I drove home, trying to beat her alarm clock, I pulled over. It felt like an outside force grabbed my hand and swerved into the nearest side street. I crawled into the backseat and ate every last bite of the new box of Pop-Tarts.

What have I done? Now I will be paying my debt to the calorie gods for the rest of the month. All alcohol and food are strictly forbidden for the foreseeable future.

I slapped myself in the face, hoping to form some sort of negative association. It never works.

Around 4 a.m. I drove to the gym, stomach full of Pop-Tarts. But once I pulled into the parking lot, I realized I had no intention of getting out. Fat Man Scoop was on Magic 102.3 playing all my favorite songs, so I drove in loops for hours waiting for daylight. I felt guilty for wasting gas, but if I went back home I'd be lured back into Alicia's pantry, so I just kept driving.

Finally the sun came up, so I pulled into the dirt lot of San Marco State Park and started running. I ignored all trail signs. I was lost in thought, thoughts about life and my disenchantment with college. It isn't what I expected. It's boring, I don't listen in class, and I can't focus.

I love going out with my sister and her friends, but my eating disorder still has a grip on me. I really miss my gaggle of high school friends, running and drinking, laughing and pranking. Overachieving predominately anorexic state champs, all hiding behind running. I got too sick my senior year and my parents told me to choose. Gain weight or quit the team. It was never a choice. I quit the team, listened to Coach Donaldson yell after me, "You're letting them all down. You're the captain. You could be top ten in the state, full ride scholarships, and you're quitting?"

He didn't know I didn't want to be the captain. I didn't care about running anymore. I couldn't travel and eat pasta dinners on the road. I could barely navigate through a Subway salad. Besides, I didn't care about running for a coach besides Coach Maddox. I was done with the team, but I wasn't done running. And now I had 3,360 calories of Alicia's Pop-Tarts to outrun.

I lost track of time. I'd set out to run at least ten miles, but no more than thirteen. I checked my pedometer at 3 p.m. and I had hit twelve miles. That should be good enough. But lost in my deep thoughts, I stopped looking for the yellow blazes to tell me where I was. I must have wandered off course. I slowed down to a walk. Besides being slightly thirsty, I was in no hurry to get back to my car. I still had five hours until sunset.

I kept walking and there were no markers to be found. I couldn't see any beaten path. I veered again, hoping maybe I would see blue blazes that could take me back to the trailhead, even if it would be further. After another hour I was devastatingly thirsty, and all I could think about was an ice cold Powerade Zero. Anything to quench my thirst. I started to run again, hoping it would get me to a drink faster.

Nothing around me had been disturbed by a human in months. All I could see were trees, light brown leaves littered on the ground, and pinecones I would have kicked if I'd had the time. Deer boldly foraged in the bushes. I heard the rustling of armadillos scurrying out of my path, and I thought back to a team run when a cottonmouth rattlesnake lurched, fangs exposed, at April Carnell's meaty calf.

What would happen if a snake bit me? Would I die a painful death, lying on a forest floor, clutching my leg as the venom reached my heart? Is that what venom does? Is it red touches black, you'll never come back? Or you're okay Jack?

I thought back to my mother screaming at me, "You're going to die of anorexia!"

The irony. Cause of death: rattlesnake.

Another hour passed and the sun set assertively. Could this be reality? Was I really going to be trapped in a forest after dark, my body discovered curled up in a tight ball, teal cobblestone shorts and a worn-out American Eagle T-shirt? If I had to be found in an outfit, I was thankful it was this one. But still, I didn't want to die. I'd lived so wrong, I had so much to atone for. My fight or flight instincts were warranted for once, and I began to scream.

"Help!" There must be some adult here, some real adult who didn't spend their morning driving down I-75 listening to Lil Boosie and lamenting a box of Pop-Tarts.

I reached a swampy field and scaled the barbed wire fence around its perimeter. The sharp edges grazed my shin to join the deeper scratches from fallen branches and bushes I'd plowed through searching for the trail. I didn't know if I was better off in the forest or the field, but changing my surroundings seemed like the best option. Changing my surroundings in hopes it will fix things is a common strategy of mine.

I heard the comforting sound of cars on a highway, so I knew I wasn't too far from civilization. I decided my best chances were being within earshot so someone could rescue me, even if it meant being bitten by a snake in a swampy field.

I tested the soggy ground directly ahead of me with a branch, making sure no snakes struck at the wood that could be my leg in another step. Finally, I beheld a beacon of hope. Off in the distance, a litter of puppies plodded along after their mother, cute little black puppies and a thick, sweet mama dog.

What breed is that? Maybe a bully breed.

I could barely make out the silhouettes. But puppies meant people, and there must have been a house I couldn't see through the dusky night.

"Help! Help! I'm lost!" Whoever owned these puppies couldn't be far.

I ran closer and froze mid-step. I'd never seen pets with such bristly fur and powerful chests. I suppressed a gasp as I realized the terrifying truth. These were feral hogs. The babies were still young, helpless, and adorable enough to make perfect displays in a pet store window. But Mama Boar was not cute. I didn't get close enough to see the wiry bristles on her snout, but her long white tusks cut through the twilight. Before she could change her path and charge toward me, I sprinted in the opposite direction, reflexively reaching my hands out behind me to protect my upper legs and ass from her wrath.

I scanned the horizon, looking for a tree to keep me off the ground, keep me from being a late-night snack for snakes, boars, and even alligators. Anything, I realized, was possible tonight. My life had become a cheap version of *Castaway*.

I grabbed a thick tree branch, pulled my body over it, climbed two more levels up, and crouched down as blackness enveloped me. And that is how I got into my current predicament, squatting in a tree and contemplating my mortality.

My primary fear, the most looming threat to my immediate life, is dehydration. Angela once taught me the rule of threes.

Three minutes without oxygen, three days without water, three weeks without food. But how does the fact that I've run for four hours, meandered for four more, and frantically sprinted for what felt like a century, factor into this equation? Nature cuts through my denial and I wonder, how will being 99 pounds alter the formula for how long I can go without food?

I think about Angela's episode summaries of *Survivorman*. It always sounds boring. Why would I care about how to survive in the wilderness? I live in an apartment. But Angela told me urine is sterile. I must take advantage of every resource at my disposal. I cup my hand and try to release into it as slowly as I can, cutting off the stream as I pause to bring my hand up to my mouth. I lose at least 30% of the fluid as it trickles down my arm, but I pray that my urine will quench my thirst. Later, as I'll recount this story to giggling girlfriends, they will ask how long it took me to resort to drinking my own pee. I did not tempt fate. Maybe two minutes.

If you are curious, and be honest with yourself, you are, pee tastes like creamy asparagus. It has a sharp aftertaste and smells like pee, shockingly. The most offensive thing about it is that it's warm. I crave cases of Powerade Zero, sugar-free grapey goodness pouring down my throat and saturating my tissues. A few handfuls of pee are not enough.

I alternate between crouching and standing. I wave my hands and wiggle strategically, swinging my head to keep the mosquitoes away. I rip my American Eagle shirt, stretch it into a tent, and drape my sweat-soaked hair over my face and neck.

The worst thing about this night is not the lightning storm that will soon drench me. It is not the hunger or the fear. It's the mosquitoes and the cold. I quiver in the darkness after being drenched by the rain, wondering if on this southern September night I will die of dehydration and exposure.

I use the backlight of my watch to illuminate the two feet I can discern below me. Leaves and branches are all I see. The rustling of deer is so constant that I don't bother to look down any more. Every five minutes I call for help, hoping a park ranger will rescue me, wrap me in a blanket, and take me back to safety.

A helicopter buzzes overhead. It lights up the swamp to my left and the forest all around me, startling the deer back into the deep recesses of the underbrush. A search team is looking for me. My parents will be mortified but at least I'll be alive.

I soon realize the helicopter is not for me. Maybe it was for a sexual predator, a serial rapist hiding out in the woods less than a mile from me. Maybe it was just taking a rich celebrity, Kanye West perhaps, to the airport. I'll never know.

Thunder claps between flashes of lightning. Rain is imminent. Thank God. Clouds of mosquitoes have been sucking my blood, buzzing in my ears, threatening my sanity. I feel ticks inch their way up my legs, trying to nestle into any crease they can find. I do my best to wipe them off before they attach, but I know I miss a few. I'm itchy, and though I try to keep moving to prevent the mosquitoes from landing, I'm running out of energy.

The clouds consolidate and thick sheets of rain pound me on the back, washing away the dirt and silencing the symphony of mosquitoes. I open my mouth and let it fill with as much rainwater as I can, washing away the urine on my tongue. I take off my shoes and let them fill with water, then bring them to my lips. I suck the water out of my salty socks, wringing them out into my mouth as I tilt my head toward the sky.

After the storm, I'm freezing. It's a crisp evening, and though in my mind I am enormous, I'm forced to ponder the benefits of padding. I shiver uncontrollably, stretching my shirt over my legs as I curl into a ball. It's a temporary reprieve from the goosebumps until mosquitoes force me to stand back up and keep dancing.

By 3 a.m., nature has shown me how small I am, a speck in the universe. I think about my Religious Studies class, a filler I am taking to remain in the Honors Program, another meaningless hoop to jump through. I have to write a paper about Tenochtitlan. I think about the Aztecs and how brutally they lived, how rigorous their training was, how little it mattered if they died. They are all dead now anyways. What would it be like to be a human sacrifice and have your brain pulled out through your nose? People have been struggling and suffering for centuries.

I think about my boyfriend, Gabe, how he's forced me to watch hours of *The Godfather*. I would rather be sitting in this tree than wake up with a horsehead next to me. Yes, my situation is not so bad, and I'm sure tomorrow I will find my way out.

My optimism is replaced with a sense of impending doom. I'm going to die and I've wasted my eighteen years on food scales and vomiting ice cream, running on treadmills, literally and figuratively.

I wonder how it will happen if things go south. If I feel my eyes droop and my body slip into a coma, my kidneys no longer able to flush me of the Pop-Tart toxins, I need a plan to avoid a protracted death. I will have to jump out of the tree and snap my own neck. When is the appropriate time to resort to such a measure? I certainly don't want to die. But a painful, drawn-out death terrifies me, which is fucking ironic for someone who has given years to anorexia.

I talk to God. God, I'm so sorry I don't believe in you. I do now. I swear I can feel you. I promise tomorrow I will wake up and go to church. I'll call Rebecca Mays and ask her to lunch, even though she snitched on me for being anorexic. Her intentions were good. If I get out of this tree I will eat normally tomorrow. I'll start volunteering again at the Saint Francis House like I did in high school and bring bread to people who can't help their hunger. I'll patch things up with my mom and I'll stop cursing. I swear to fucking God. Just please help me. I love you God. I'll stop underage drinking. I'll meditate like Rachel wants me to. Just please don't let me die, not like this.

God listens but I do not. I renege on our deal. The next morning, I climb out of the tree, pick up a fallen branch, and beat it on the ground in front of me. I'm still rightfully paranoid about snakes. Large magnolia leaves filled with rainwater form miniature cups, and I take advantage of every opportunity to flood my parched body with water. I don't want to overexert myself. I'm running on foot-water and urine. But I'm also racing time. I jog in a random direction, hoping to get lucky.

At 10 a.m. I happen upon a photo booth (I know very little about hunting and don't realize it's actually a deer feeder.)

Why is there a photo booth filled with bird seed? Should I take a handful of seeds for sustenance? No, seeds are full of fat. One handful of seeds could undo God knows how many miles I ran yesterday.

You can plead with God all you want and stare death in the face in the middle of a forest, but if your training partner is anorexia, don't expect to magically eat bird seed just because it's a special occasion.

Off in the distance I see something unmistakable, human life and a golf cart. Two talkative southern hunters deliver me back to safety and inform me that I am no longer in the running section of the park. I have crossed into the state preserve, where hunting is allowed.

"Yeah, you're lucky we didn't shoot you. We coulda' thought you were a deer pokin' around that deer feeder like that," the golf cart driver tells me. "We should call the papers. Do you need to go to the hospital, honey?"

I know I'm a mess. My hair is arranged over my face like the girl in *The Ring*, an improvised mosquito net. There's dirt caked under my nails and I'm sopping wet. I picture the newspapers and am immediately mortified. My parents can't read about this.

I lost my car keys in the woods, never to be recovered, so I call my sister to pick me up. My sister, simultaneously amused, shocked, and not surprised at all, beholds the spectacle that is me.

"Oh my God, Jen. Should we go to the hospital to get you checked out?" I have no intention of explaining that bill to my parents.

"Okay, well let's go to 53rd Street Deli and get some pancakes. You must be starving," my sister suggests as she cranks the engine.

She knows I don't eat pancakes, but she must think that under these circumstances, after having a near death experience, the rules will be lifted for just for a moment. I picture Rebecca Mays and me mending our relationship over pita bread and salmon. Me going to church luncheons. These were adrenaline-filled promises. I will do all of those things, but I just need to stabilize. I need a day of counting, because I am still in a caloric surplus.

"Natalie, I just want to go home and take a shower." I do want to take a shower, but the truth is God's face is fading now and the tabulations are resuming in my mind. I will start my new ways tomorrow, totally abandon this eating disorder and see the light, but today I need to count and make up for the Pop-Tarts. I refuse to admit it even to myself, but there will be no Rebecca Mays. There will be no church luncheons. And there will damned sure be no pancakes, because even after God has doused me with rain and ticks, pelting me with warnings, I know deep down that if I were to sit in a diner and stare down a plate of pancakes swimming in syrup, I would get the same exact feeling as when I saw that Mama Boar.

Swimming Pools

My first semester of college, my sister has not yet moved to Washington, D.C. to pursue her political career. I realize at this point in my saga I come across as quite peculiar, but for some reason Natalie has never hesitated to include me in her social circle. If you can overlook the fact that I do not eat in front of people and retreat into the abyss of my apartment four times a day to feast, hang upside down like a bat, or hide frozen corpses in my freezer (I assume these are the scenarios people imagine), I enjoy socializing. I have enough self-awareness to censor my inner douche bag, so long as my sister is around to prevent me from wearing cubic zirconia earrings five sizes too big.

So while the Pop-Tart binges and nights in the forest constantly hum in the background, the soundtrack to my life, I do find a sense of collegiate normalcy. I effortlessly make the

Dean's List, wishing academic woes were the extent of my adversity. I develop a reputation for liking "The Vod", and though my eating habits are in shambles, drinking alcohol is relatively safe in my eyes. I join my sister and her friends, perfect girls she met in her sorority, for raucous nights on the town. Like the student council of our high school, I assume I am a legacy pick, only allowed to join this elite group because I am the younger sister of a cool girl. My sister doesn't need to try. She naturally has fashion sense, good hair, and attracts men as if they are dogs and she has bacon stuffed in her pockets.

Her friends are girls like that, not girls with Moon Boots. Girls who join sororities and book cruises for Spring Break. But they show me a normal world that is equally as fun as bouncing in an anti-gravity atmosphere and filling bathtubs with milk and Corn Pops. When Natalie moves away, I assume her posse will ditch her weirdo sister. To my shock, they continue to invite me out with them, and I become overwhelmed trying to keep up with their busy social calendars. Four years younger, I am a source of entertainment, always vowing to not make a sloppy spectacle of myself until someone sets a shot glass in front of me. I eye the glass of clear vodka, as innocent as water, and think back drunkenly to the four bags of peanuts I accidentally ate that morning. Then I pour the liquor down in haste as I suppress a gag, drowning out the reminder that I am out of control with peanuts. My plan to starve now that I am no longer under my parents' supervision is failing miserably, and instead I put on the

Freshman 10, which looks more like the Freshman 40 to me in the mirror.

Gabe is my boyfriend. I meet him at a bar called Froggy's and we dance raunchily to Usher. *Love in this Club.*

"Do you want to go to the bathroom?" he whispers in my ear as the music drowns out the drunken squeals of undergrad debauchery.

"No, I just went," I respond, missing my cue to have sticky urine bathroom sex. I am still holding on to my purity at this point, more from lack of interest than morality.

Gabe takes me on a proper bowling date the next weekend. I am disappointed when I see him through my peephole with sober eyes. I try not to be. But despite being a cute frat boy, despite being the type of guy my sister and her friends approve of, there is no meaty veiny edginess to him. His ears are unpierced, no diamonds. No tattoos. He loves Tarantino movies, and I try to find this as desirable as he seems to think it is. He reads Voltaire and studied abroad. He speaks two languages and is learning a third. I want Gabe to be my type, but I never tell him I have an eating disorder, and this creates a gulf so large that he may as well still be abroad even as we sit next to each other under the Christmas lights he keeps up year-round.

By the time Valentine's Day rolls around, I have taken the cockroach exhibit off of my gallery wall in defeat, finally accepting the endless cycle of binge-try unsuccessfully to purge-exercise. Gabe wants to cook me a taco dinner. I tell him I have a huge exam to cram for, which might be true. But really I have many miles to swim and run, and that is after an appointment at the Student Health Care Center. I finally realize that being 18 with no period is likely not healthy, and I am scheduled to see a doctor to discuss my options.

Gabe meets me in Kensington Plaza after my Abnormal Psychology class and gives me a box of chocolates to commemorate the holiday. Before he has even loaded his bike on the front of the city bus to begin his journey home, I've devoured the entire heart-shaped box. Then I go to my appointment, the first time I will be honest with a doctor now that I am legally an adult.

I'm 99 pounds at this point, and the fact that my doctor considers this slightly underweight tells me all I need to know. She is in the Obesity Mafia, my anorexic mind's version of the Illuminati. Doctors have been trying to lure me into chubbiness my entire life, and I have never trusted them.

"This is a serious problem, Jen. Your body fat has been too low for too long, and your body can't make estrogen. Estrogen is what makes your bones strong. You need to get a bone density scan."

The results are devastating. Normal bone density is a T-score of 0. Most strong, young people have something slightly above 0, perhaps a +0.5, and some football players and bodybuilding men have scores as high as +2. My score is -2.9, equivalent to most women in their eighties.

How could this be? I have always taken calcium, always exercised, always done almost everything just right...the only thing I didn't do was get a period. Rebecca Mays' mom was right. My Achilles tendon menstruation was not enough. I am much too clever to have something like this happen to me.

This news is a major bummer, and once I get home I set my sights on extra-cushioned running shoes. It would be terrible to get a stress fracture and not be able to run for six weeks. This is the extent of the importance I place on my osteoporosis diagnosis. I never imagine one day it will become an all-consuming acid that will etch away my mind.

One day I look at the blank wall over my computer that used to be so hopeful, so full of cockroaches that acknowledged I could stop bingeing any day. I realize that now my goal has to be weight gain, and it can't be muscle. Only the estrogen stored in body fat has any hope of helping my bones.

Gabe breaks up with me over the phone as I rest between sets on the tricep pulley. Something about how I'm never available, but I was only half listening. My bequeathed sorority friends still invite me out all the time, but I start to abuse my prescription for Concerta, depending on the stimulant to magnify the vodka enough for me to get hammered on fewer calorie-laden drinks.

Everything feels out of control and I vow to stop drinking, but every time I go out I get shitfaced. I pin the issue on alcohol because I know that the true issue is food, which for me is a much more unavoidable daily temptation. One night my friend Michelle invites me over for a movie night. Everyone else brings wine, but I bring vodka because the sugar in wine scares me. Michelle has a bottle of absinthe on top of her fridge that nobody else likes. Because my sloppiness is seen as typical of undergrad students at Brighton, everyone laughs as I take shots while they sip wine.

I'm too drunk to drive home so I take a cab, and as I wobble upstairs my Creepy Downstairs Neighbor invites me to come in. I have on a blue hairband. He tells me he has an allergy to phenylalanine, something in diet soda, and he has a twin brother. Later, as I try to recall his name, this is all I will be left with.

The next morning I wake up on my own floor and my headband is gone. So is my underwear. I'm still in my blue flowered sundress. I immediately wonder if I have AIDS. If I have no underwear, did we have sex? I knock on his door and ask if I should get tested. He says no, he wore a condom. I ask for my hairband back.

I realize my out-of-controlness is everything from eating to drinking to now sleeping with Creepy Downstairs Neighbor. I waited eighteen years to have sex and my second partner was the guy downstairs who once asked me to stop stomping as I learned the Soulja Boy dance. I'm disgusting.

I call my sister after chugging half a handle of vodka. I talk to her as I stumble through an empty field behind my apartment complex, and I can tell she stays on the phone out of concern. Once we hang up, I knock on Creepy Downstairs

Neighbor's door. I want to know his name, want to know how old he is, want to know something about this person I just gave so much to. His roommate answers instead so I stumble back upstairs.

I look at my bottle of Prozac that I know for sure is not working and I take a handful. Then a few Concerta and Tylenol PM washed down with calcium citrate and half a bottle of multivitamins. To this day I'm not sure if this episode is an attempt to hurt myself or flood my body with nutrition. If I want to hurt myself, it clearly is not a lasting intention because I immediately call Angela, slurring, and tell her I am scared I overdosed. She takes me to the emergency room where they pump my stomach. I wake up with both of my parents by my bedside and a security guard outside my door. When I ask to go to the bathroom, he escorts me and explains I have been 5150'd, a mental hold.

I hear my dad pleading with a nurse to not transport me by ambulance to the psychiatric ward, that it had just been a cry for help. Maybe he was right. But whenever I think of this episode I'm reminded of a time in middle school when I lost control rollerblading down a steep slope. I could see cars zooming at the bottom of the hill and I grasped frantically at branches to stop my momentum, clutching for anything to stop the cars from flattening me, anything to stop my free fall.

I Must Be On Somethin'

Kyle and I meet in the middle of the night shortly after this traumatic episode. I'm wearing a camo student council T-shirt, Nike Tempo running shorts with a Cardinals logo, and no makeup, the latter of which I'm acutely aware of from the moment he approaches me. He's on the floor team of Sanford Health and Fitness, sporting the uniform royal blue button-down shirt and black slacks. His button nose and Neanderthal brow ridge remind me of Matt Damon, but with light blonde hair. He looks like an attractive frog. I can't tell what his body looks like underneath the blue button-down, but I see enough to know that he is athletic, and possibly a former runner.

He approaches me as I adjust the notches on the lumbar back extension machine, which later in our relationship becomes infinitely ironic.

"Do you need help with that? Here, let me adjust the leg pad." He moves a few levers and gestures for me to sit down. I pretend to be oblivious and eternally grateful for his assistance.

"I used to run cross country and my back would always kill me at the end of races. I started doing this machine and my back pain vanished by the end of the season." He shifts from one foot to the other as he speaks.

I wonder if this is true or just a fabricated story to fill the dead air. Then Kyle launches into a detailed tutorial about how to perform the exercise. I tune him out after several seconds.

How many laps do I need to swim after this? Could I skip the yogurt at breakfast tomorrow and go home early tonight?

I keep a smile painted on, not wanting to seem uninterested. I am very interested, but not in the machine. Kyle's babble seems like nerves, and I'm flattered.

"We should go for a run or do lunch. My name's Kyle." He takes a slip of paper from beside the suggestion box and writes down his number. I do the same, wondering if I am supposed to give him mine as well. It seems redundant, but rude not to reciprocate. I save him to my contacts and try to hide my bashfulness.

I accidentally call Kyle more than thirty times in the weeks that follow. For an inexplicable reason, when I call anyone at all, my caller ID displays an outgoing call to Kyle. He never calls back, and I assume he has written me off as a mentally unstable stalker. I am not a stalker.

No, my obsessions tend to revolve around more obscure topics. My follow-up bone density scan shows that positive thinking and half-assed attempts at weight gain are not sufficient, and my -2.9 T-score is now a -3.2. I plug my diagnosis into Google and am assaulted with images of old women hunched over like Quasimoto. They look like my grandmother, shorter each year with her stomach protruding in the worst of ways. Her spine is permanently deformed like a big letter S, her vertebrae crushed like dominos, pushing her stomach out because it has nowhere else to go. I can't imagine a worse disease for someone with a phobia of protruding stomachs, and I spend many sleepless nights reading horror stories that hijack my brain.

If my spine were ever to fracture like Grammy's, my world would be over. Luckily, I quickly craft a solution. I'll commit suicide if that happens. If I ever break my spine or get a hunchback, I'll experience one painful pull of a trigger, then POOF- problem solved.

But I have years to ensure this will never happen and my osteoporosis stays a silent disease.

I will get my estrogen levels up, which will give me a period. If I can get my period then I can build my bones and stop peeing them out. Angela promises me that once I officially hit puberty she will throw me a Princess Menses party like I'm a thirteen-year-old girl with very progressive parents.

I try acupuncture and drink raw cow's milk each morning. Every night before bed, I gag down a large bowl of raw kale for the plant-based calcium. I dump cod liver oil into my oatmeal. I eat one raw egg a day and three prunes for no good reason other than to seal my favorability with Mother Nature so she will make it rain in my ovaries. I register on the National Osteoporosis Foundation forum boards as J-bones, desperate to glean any knowledge that will help me prevent a hunchback.

I scour the internet for steroids, because along with big muscles, steroids make thick bones. I locate a clinical trial in Boston for girls my age with anorexia and osteoporosis, because unfortunately if you have anorexia and are reading this, you probably have it too. During this trial I'm expected to take two subcutaneous injections of IGF-1 a day, even though there is a 50% chance I'm in the unfortunate placebo group that injects sugar water instead. IGF-1 is a hormone bodybuilders use to get bigger, but in the microdoses I take, it is supposed to regulate my hormones and catch me up on the eight years I lost peeing out bone while other girls laid down a nice, strong foundation of skeletal (and mental) health.

For the next year, my thighs and stomach are covered in tiny bruises from the needle sticks, and every few weeks I pee all day into a container resembling a gas tank so that the researchers can measure how much bone I'm losing. It's fun to lug a duffel bag of urine onto the city bus, in a cooler to keep it cold, or sit with it beside me in lecture halls as I listen to my Chem 2 professor discuss strong bases and acids. This unit strikes close to home because I basically want strong acid, or something to get me away from my pee-lugging, hormone-shooting existence. Even worse, I feel ridiculous in my new 103-pound body, the weight the experts in Boston told me was the minimum for any hope of a period. I make my back muscles so strong at the gym that I wonder if the IGF-1 actually is working like a steroid.

Every three months I get a new bone density scan and every three months I see my bones get worse. I drop out of the trial. It's a waste of money to fly to Boston when I'm clearly the unfortunate control group shooting up vials of sugar water as I watch my -3.2 turn to -3.3 to -3.5. I also drop the 103 pounds, which I'll get to later.

I find a local expert, Dr. Styles, MD PHD. At first, his receptionist tells me he is not accepting new patients, so I write him an earnest letter. I attach my bone density scans and confide I am terrified of becoming a hunchback and if he could find it in his schedule, I would do anything to be his patient. He calls me the next day, and when I meet him he's nothing like I pictured.

He's old, with a pornstar mustache and a white coat. He's matter-of-fact, kind, and reminds me a lot of my dad, which is slightly creepy since he is also my gynecologist. He scans my uterus like a spelunker in a cave and informs me there will be no Princess Menses party or baby shower in my future. My hypothalamus and pituitary gland are permanently out of communication after years of being toyed with. All my acupuncture and weight gain and IGF-1 might as well have been snake oil, because my uterus is about as dysfunctional as my brain.

"Jen, you aren't going to get a period. It's unlikely you'll be able to have kids because there is no lining for an embryo to attach to. You have very low estrogen and it's not something you can get naturally at this point. I'm going to start you on hormone replacement therapy."

Hormone replacement therapy is like birth control, but instead of preventing pregnancy, it just adds extra hormones to my body through a clear patch I wear on my ass. It is usually reserved for postmenopausal women, which is the excuse my insurance company uses each month to make me pay the full cost.

This is tough, but the next part destroys me. He gives me a follow-up bone density scan and calls me later with the results. Though I didn't think it was possible, my bones have gotten even worse.

"You have no bone left to lose. Let's see what the hormones do, but we really need to get you on prescription osteoporosis medication. Keep lifting weights and doing the elliptical, because strong muscles will help your bones. But running and jumping are too high-impact for someone with your T-scores." The way he explains impact is that if one foot is still on the ground, it's low-impact and okay to do. If both feet leave the ground, it's high-impact and too much of a jolt.

I hang up the phone and grab my flats, lightweight racing shoes from my high school track days. I blast Tupac, *Thugz*

Mansion. His lyrics about death bring me hope that there's an escape, but not in a healthy way.

That's what I'll do. If I ever get a hunchback, I'll hold that 9 and I'll off myself. It will be that simple. I have to figure out what a 9 is first.

At the time, this is such an obvious solution. I don't consider that this would kill my family, Angela, and the new dog I adopted. I also know deep down that my odds of getting a hunchback at my age are pretty low. But it comforts me to know that if down the road I did, there's an exit plan. It's not like I'll have kids to stick around for.

Still, I really do not want to die. I must devote my life to the strongest spine ever. But first, one last mile. I park my car at my old high school track. My last mile is faster than I ever ran at a track meet. I finally break 5:30 and nobody is there to see it. And that was the last time I ever ran.

I realize gaining weight actually doesn't really help my bones anymore because everything in my body is now artificial, from hormones to bone density to even my brain chemistry, controlled by antidepressants and antipsychotics. There's something a bit unnerving about this realization, about realizing that by the age of twenty I have irreversibly fucked up so many things and that every major system in my body now needs to be exogenously controlled.

The silver lining to this period of time is that I decide to pursue my goal of attending physical therapy school. As soon as I have my Doctorate of Physical Therapy, I will know exactly what to do to make sure I never have to hold that 9 in my hand and blow my brains out because I'm a hunchback.

Rehab

I may never teach my uterus to shed its lining, but I do manage to teach myself to purge everything in my stomach, not just ice cream. It is arduous at first, not like in the movies where a little girl decides she's fat and daintily purges her mom's chicken before bed. At first, I have to stick my fingers down my throat for minutes at a time only to bring up a small amount of food, then repeat the process over and over for up to an hour. I leave the bathroom, exhausted and thankful for a clear airway not blocked off by my own fingers. I'm incredibly jealous of girls who don't need to use their fingers, a wish that will one day come true and ruin my life.

I still absorb some calories at this haphazard phase of purging, so I perform exercise punishment to prevent weight gain. I call my self-torture plan "3-5-7." The day after a binge-purge episode, I allot myself 300 calories of mostly tuna and brussels sprouts. The following day two packets of oatmeal are added for a total of 500 calories. And by the third day, as long as I maintained the triple workouts the previous days, I add a family-size bag of broccoli. The rest of the week I can eat full calories but still must perform exercise penance. Not being able to run makes this rather inefficient, and many days my classes get in the way of hours on the elliptical, in the pool, or on a stationary bike. I lose a massive amount of weight through this ritual, all performed to guarantee I do not become a fat bulimic.

Rachel urges me to get inpatient help, something which I have been threatened with since I was sixteen. The impetus for me finally going was Rachel's client, fresh out of Maravilla, coming in to tell me about her experience. She says all the therapists there are like mirror images of Rachel and it changed her life. She was allowed to hike, and there are gym passes if you follow the treatment plan. Rachel's client doesn't look fat at all. So I tell my parents I have an exercise addiction, book a ticket to Arizona, and blast Young Money's *Bedrock* on my optimistic drive to the airport.

A woman with flawless olive skin picks me up in a big white van. It reminds me of the vans at Oakwood, a facility I volunteer at that houses adults with profound intellectual disabilities.

What kind of a place is this?

The woman and I make small talk on the drive from the airport and she feels more like a peer than anyone in an authority position. I quickly learn that she is a CA, or Community Attendant. CAs are usually employees paid minimum wage to watch over residents, fulfilling a role that lies somewhere between babysitter and Corrections Officer. A major perk for most of them is the free cuisine prepared by chefs, so long as they are willing to eat surrounded by sobbing residents.

As soon as we arrive at the facility, a nurse takes my picture outside against a brick wall and tells me, "It's amazing how different and healthy you'll look when you check out. The before and after pictures here are amazing."

I think I already look amazing.

It's almost Christmas, and there's a tree in the common area. To the left is a huge table with placemats covered in motivational phrases like **Be strong** or **You'll get through this**. Just as I begin to wheel my suitcase to my room, I'm told I need to be searched. Two staffers pat me down and ask me to empty my pockets. All of my gum is placed in a Ziplock bag labeled **Contraband**. So is my self-tanner.

"Wait, I can't tan?" Being pale makes me picture Jake and his mayonnaise, so I am slightly perturbed.

"That's body-image oriented. You're here to focus on your mental health," says one of the CAs as he rifles through my clothes. This makes sense I suppose, and I want to be compliant. They confiscate the celebrity magazines from the airport and all of my razors. I learn that I will be allowed to shave once they trust I do not self-harm. All of my multivitamins are dumped because the bottle isn't sealed, and my exercise resistance bands are put in separate **Contraband** bags. This I have an issue with.

"Wait! I have an inflamed bursa in my knee! My pes anserine bursitis! I need those bands!" I am more concerned that I will no longer be able to activate my gluteus medius and will leave treatment with a floppy pancake ass. But I watch in defeat as all of my contraband is taken to a storage shed and locked up for the remainder of my stay.

My roommate is relieved to see me. She's a sweet, peppy blonde here over Christmas break at Arizona State University. Her sorority sisters call her Jazz.

"The girl before you was psychotic. Seriously unhinged. Her name was Marcy and she had two personalities, no lie. She was old, like 36."

Marcy had been kicked out because she hid string cheese in her hair and hoarded it under her bed to chew and spit after lights-out. She took the dollops of butter she was supposed to eat and rubbed them into her skin to erase the evidence.

Maybe I am not severe enough for inpatient care.

"So what's the exercise like here? How often can we go to the gym?" I ask. Rachel's client promised that gym time was guaranteed.

Jazz informs me that because it is Christmas break, gym time is replaced by yoga, but at least once a week. I do the math in my head. If I'm here for three weeks, that is horrible but worth recovery I suppose. I know that I have an addiction to exercise and I truly want to stop.

Jazz looks me over once and says, "There's no way they'll clear you to do anything though. Maybe mindful walking but I doubt it."

Mindful walking is miserable. To eliminate any exercise fix walking might provide, mindful walking is loitering through a labyrinth so slowly I almost lose my balance. I'm supposed to examine my inner thoughts, but instead I clinch every muscle in my body in an attempt to feel some sort of burn. I pin my hopes on our camping trip, where us inpatient girls will meet up with the women in the halfway house for a mountain retreat. The halfway house residents have already graduated from inpatient and can do wild things like walk to the store unsupervised and cook their own meals.

My first week is relatively easy. My dietician is booked up due to staff shortages, so I'm put on the meal plan that guarantees I won't get "refeeding syndrome," a fatal shift in electrolytes that anorexics can develop if they eat too much food after months of starvation. This meal plan is barely enough for me to maintain my weight, so though I hate not being able to exercise, I'm not frantic... yet.

Three days before Christmas, we take a winding mountain pathway to a cabin owned by the facility, and most of the staff comes along. It's freezing cold and I wear a blue beanie that Jazz says makes me look like a cancer patient. I think it makes me look like a thug, and I hope it will send a message to the staff that I am hearty enough to partake in all activities. Our first night, food is laid buffet style on a plastic folding luncheon table. As I go through the line to serve my plate and have it checked off by the supervising CA, my dietician hands me a new, laminated card. A new meal card. It doubles my previous meal plan, and Jen II emerges.

"No, fuck no. What the fuck? I'm doing well. That's so many starches. Nobody can eat that much. What, I'm just supposed to eat two potatoes like that's nothing? That's preposterous! I have rights!"

My nails dig deeply into my neck skin, leaving raised slash marks that prevent me from ever earning the privilege to shave my legs. The next morning I get dressed for the hike, hoping that if I'm fully dressed they will decide it's convenient enough to bring me along. A CA tells me I will stay behind with the cleaning crew for nature therapy. This is a euphemism for sitting in the cabin begging to help mop, but being told this is too strenuous and an excuse to burn calories.

"How is hiking exercise?" I ask the CA indignantly.

"You have to be here at least two weeks and gain weight to do any activity beyond mindful walking."

I am used to up to six hours of exercise a day and I'm crawling out of my skin. The rest of the camping trip is excruciating, and because it is Christmas break, many of my therapy appointments are canceled. Jazz graduates and I'm simultaneously lonely and jealous. She never had to gain weight, only stop purging.

In the third week, I snap. After three weeks of being yelled at if I stand compulsively or fidget in my chair, I lose sight of the big picture and forget my purpose for being there. To not be allowed any physical outlet is the worst claustrophobia imaginable. Myopia is intense in inpatient treatment, and I discover over the years that promises I make to myself about the monumental importance of getting my life back are eclipsed by panic, terror... and cowardice.

I say the magic words. "I want to go home."

Suddenly all the staff is available. Christmas can wait. I'm taken to a large conference room where Dyna, the CEO, who must spend most of her paycheck on Botox while I can't use self-tanner, tells me that if I leave against medical advice there's a risk my insurance won't pay. She tells me I can't use a phone. That I don't have that privilege.

"I'm being held captive. Get me the fuck out of here. I have rights! I have rights!"

"You have nothing to go home to. You can't exercise there either, sweetie. Your mom canceled your gym membership. The gym won't let you come back."

The first time in my life that I surrendered, the minute I left town, my mom got me kicked out of the gym against Rachel's advice. Once the gym saw how many check-ins a day I used and my mom told them I was anorexic, they no longer felt it was worth the liability until I produced a doctor's note. In my mind, I couldn't afford to sit helplessly in Arizona. I had to get home and straighten things out.

If I could go back in time, I would beg myself to stay. I would tell myself the most important investment I will ever make is to stay an extra month, no matter how imperfect Maravilla is and how angry I am at my mom. I would try as hard as I could to convince myself that eating disorders just get worse when you treat them with kid gloves, and that everyone around me will progress in their lives and I will stay stuck. I wish I had been braver and realized I was rebelling against myself.

They allow me to call Rachel. She tries to talk me down as I scream that I'll be homeless and pawn all my clothes, all my jewelry, just for a plane ticket home. That I'll do anything in the world, just get me the fuck out of here. I'll sit in a tree and drink my pee for the rest of my life. I don't consider the fact that the most valuable possession to my name is a pretzel necklace with cubic zirconia adornments from Target.

Still, the next day I refuse to eat. Though they threaten to have me committed to a hospital and put on a feeding tube, I call their bluff and am finally allowed to fly home. My parents and I will not speak for months.

I move in with Angela and her family while I get my feet under me. I gain some of the weight I need to, and as badly as I portray Maravilla, my exercise addiction truly was cured. To this day, I never over-exercise. I love the gym. I love activity. But never again will I use it as a tool for weight loss.

My eating disorder had convinced me I would get fat if I didn't exercise. Three weeks of extreme rest exposed its lies. Despite the lack of therapy, despite the anger at my mom for intervening when I had already surrendered, to this day I am thankful for my time at Maravilla because it did fix one symptom of my eating disorder. Unfortunately, many more were left to conquer.

Below is a Christmas rap I wrote but never sent to my sister, found in my journal from treatment, a journal that was later confiscated for being full of "unhelpful thoughts."

So I'm laying here in bed and it's been a long day
I don't know where to start because I've got so much to say
I'm on Day 7 here in Tucson, Arizona
And it hasn't been easy man, of that I gotta warn ya
There are 8 girls here living under one roof
And at first I felt out of place, like a big goof
But I'm opening up and doing OK now
And they haven't made me fat like a big old spotted cow
The food is delicious and it's all organic
Everyone has breakdowns and our shrink is the mechanic
Ranya's the oldest because now she's 42
But we have so much in common, she's anorexic too!
She was forced to come here after she slit her wrists
She broke her pelvis in a fall and tried not to exist
She's funny though, and sweet, but can be a drama queen
She'll cry if a staffer makes her eat an extra bean
Nara is up next and she's 39 years old

At first I didn't like her cuz she seemed so icy cold
She's a nympho alcoholic, and also a rape victim
And she has to stay 6 months, sentenced by the court system
I don't know details but she tried to kick the bucket
She was 79 pounds and decided to say fuck it
Now she's on welfare cuz she's too messed up to work
I guess going that low in weight just makes you go berserk
Last weekend we went camping and I couldn't go for hikes
They think I'm sickly here, which I can't say that I like
They're really big on seeing this whole thing as a disease
And a man stands by the shower while I say the ABCs
This may sound creepy but I know I'd purge in there
So I guess some of these rules actually turn out to be fair
I really miss you guys, Mom, Dad, and Abby
And I can't wait to get home and live the rest of my life happy
No matter what happens in life I know you will be there
You're my best friend, older sister, and big old Snuggle Bear!

How To Love

Two years elapse from our first interaction and I don't see Kyle again. I assume he has switched shifts, possibly to escape my harassment. My exercise addiction is gone and is now entirely replaced with self-induced vomiting, so even if he does still work the overnight shift at Sanford Health and Fitness, there's little risk I'll see him.

Then one afternoon, Kyle comes back into my life. But instead of the spry young runner I remembered, a muscular bodybuilder with the same Matt Damon frogface cuts in front of me as I approach the ellipticals. My mouth opens in disbelief. He's gained at least forty pounds of muscle, veins bulging out of thick forearms. He reminds me of a bear on a bicycle, his frame threatening to buckle under the weight of his brawn. I'm instantly attracted, and I wince in embarrassment about the barrage of accidental phone calls.

To my shock, a few days later Kyle sends me a text.

Hey, it was really good running into you. I know this is two years too late, but would you want to get sushi sometime?

Sushi is a meal that Rachel and I have practiced almost every month since I returned from residential treatment. It doesn't always go smoothly, and I'm still in a delicate place in my recovery. I question whether I am truly ready to date, and knowing Kyle is an option makes it even more frustrating. I don't know how to handle the dilemma, so I ignore him. I begrudgingly accept that my dinner will be a chicken fried rice Lean Cuisine and a sweet potato eaten alone for the rest of my life.

For the next two weeks, I can't stop thinking about Kyle. I don't want to jeopardize my recovery, but I can see him being my future husband and it hurts to let that pass me by. It's a time sensitive situation because I know that eventually Kyle will ask another girl out. A girl who doesn't have an eating disorder, a girl who can get sushi without thinking, a girl who will let him sleep over and cook breakfast in the morning.

I'm jealous of Angela, how she can fall head over heels for a man and go out to dinner without reservation, no pun intended. I'm stuck in a relationship with food, and when I'm not plunging head first into my addiction, I'm trapped within the rigid walls of recovery. My life will always be like swimming in water wings, never able to enjoy the surf.

At my weekly appointment with Rachel, I'm defiant the entire session, questioning whether going to inpatient treatment was a waste of time and wondering if it's too late for me to change. I don't mention Kyle or how hurt I am that he's just beyond my reach. It kills me to know that if I were to send one simple text, I could get to know this person and it could lead to something special. I want to sabotage it before it begins and prove to myself that there is no decision to be made. I'm far too damaged to get into a relationship. I want to lose control and wallow in the hopelessness of my circumstances.

My parents are away, and though we are not on speaking terms since my return from Maravilla, I run my finger along the blade of their spare key. They live less than a mile from Rachel's office, so I decide to go over and look through old photo albums of family memories before my eating disorder tore us apart. I walk into the foyer and am greeted by a framed photo, a chubby girl in a gymnastics uniform with a gummy smile and matching hair band.

How am I that same person? I reach out to touch her, but the glass is too thick. *I'm sorry. I'm sorry that I've done this to you, that I spent all the money you saved on binge food. That I never went after your dream of being a veterinarian because I'm too scared. That a baby doll is the closest thing to a baby you'll ever have.*

I walk straight into my parents' kitchen and open up their pantry. It's full of bran cereal and crackers, food I wouldn't typically binge on. But I do anyway. I get my Biggie CD out of my car and put it in their stereo. I already know what song I want to play. *Suicidal Thoughts.*

The lyrics magnify the despair I already feel. There's no way out of this cage. I'm in an abusive relationship and I'm the abuser. I can't eat until I get permission, I'm constantly paying off debts from massive binges, I dropped out of rehab, and I'm the black sheep of my family.

I shovel food in my mouth, gulping it down with desperation. I pull out a photo album. There's me in a Purple Dragons jersey with a basketball under my arm and my dad kneeling behind me. We're happy. I never thought that I would end up so miserable. I keep flipping through old photos, my sister and I digging a mud pit, me clinging to her on her first day of middle school, us at Disney World posing with Goofy. Me blowing out the candles on my eleventh birthday cake. This is the last birthday I'll have where cake will just be cake.

I purge once and lose the gamble. The chemicals purging releases are like rolling a dice. I either get high off of the emptiness or plunge into the darkest mood imaginable. As I get older and more entrenched in my disease my lows become lower. Senseless episodes of rage are not uncommon, where I irrationally destroy everything in my path and take out my frustration on inanimate objects around me.

I slam a lamp against the wall, shattering it and breaking a light socket in the process. I go to the garage, open a case of my dad's Amber Bock, and begin chugging. I rummage through my parents' medicine cabinet and wash a fistful of sleeping pills down with another beer, and then jump in the pool, fully clothed. Still soaking wet, I go for another round, trying to roll the dice again in hopes that this time it will go better.

In the midst of my drunken destruction, I text Kyle. **Hey, I'm really sorry but I'm just getting this text. I lost my phone charger. But I would love to get dinner tomorrow :)** Blurry eyes and fat fingers, I proofread the text several times before I press send. I know if it's not tomorrow, I'll back out.

He replies in less than two minutes, and a date is made for Kabooki Sushi the next evening. I'm momentarily pleased. But then I look around me. I go to my parents' full-length mirror, the same mirror I body-checked in for the first seventeen years of my life. *Who would ever want me? Who would want this train wreck?*

I return to the garage and get another beer, opening a new case. In my haste to drown out my self-pity, I forget how to open it. I tug and tug, but stop before I pull off my fingernails. Impatiently, I put the bottle between my two front teeth and snap the top off, along with half of my front tooth. If I could go back to that moment and tell Younger Me anything... I would tell her it was a twist top.

I wake up the next morning and the first thing I do is feel for my tooth. Was that a drunken hallucination? It, in fact, was not. I look in the mirror and it's worse than I thought. The tooth is jagged, and it hangs down like a fang.

"Angela, does it really look that bad?" I ask once I get home. I want to convince myself I'm just being self-conscious.

"I mean, there's no way to look at you and not notice it. I'll put it that way." Angela is being kind.

I text Kyle, disappointed that my plan to sabotage the date was such a success.

Hey, I may have to cancel our date. I fell down my stairs and hit my tooth on a railing.

His response is not dismissive. It's chatty. He tells me a story about getting caught in a leg press at the gym, which further confirms that he's a meathead and will be more understanding of my obsession with calories. It's enough for me to change my mind.

If you promise not to laugh at me, we could still go. I just look really bad right now.

He promises not to laugh. And he doesn't until a month into our relationship, when he tells me the fact I left the house looking so utterly ridiculous had impressed him.

I'm so nervous when I see him outside of the restaurant that I don't notice he forgot to make reservations. The thought of eating in front of him, and with half a front tooth, is all the space I have available in my mind. I do my best not to smile with my mouth open, but within a few minutes I forget. Thankfully there's another sushi place within walking distance, so we make awkward conversation as we relocate our date.

He talks a lot. That's the first thing I notice about Kyle. He can turn a two minute story into a ten minute chronicle. But it doesn't annoy me at all. I actually appreciate it because it gives me a chance to chew my food and not have to think about how to coordinate talking at the same time, or whether I have seaweed stuck in one of my thirty-one-and-a-half teeth.

My next observation is that I misjudged his dedication to nutrition. He orders three deep fried rolls, slathers them in mayonnaise-based spicy sauce, and washes them down with a craft beer. I look at the veins popping out of his forearms. Could he be on steroids? Fat blocking pills? I'm perplexed. I wonder if he has a six-pack.

Still, I feel like I can't share with him, like I'm censoring myself. His nervousness helps me let my guard down, but I try to mimic what my sister, normal and desirable, would say in response to his questions.

"What kind of music do you like?" he asks.

For the life of me I cannot think of one non-rap musician. I want to seem like Natalie, not me. "Train. I love Train."

He nods in approval. "They're pretty good. What's your favorite song of theirs?"

I fumble over my words, nervously shredding my napkin and balling it up between my fingers, poking the grains of rice on my plate and mushing them beneath my wooden chopsticks. "I like all of them. All of their songs are so good."

Much later in our relationship, he will tell me watching me eat sushi that night was like watching someone dissect a rat.

I leave the date feeling uneasy, but not because I don't like him. It's because I do. I want to get hurt. I want to like someone enough to get hurt, enough to lie in bed mourning the loss of our love and drowning my sorrows in wine the way Angela does. I don't like him like that. But if anybody can lift the spell that's been cast on me, damning me to a life where every bite is a guilt-laden morsel of physiologically-essential torture, it's Kyle.

Love The Way You Lie

"When can I see you again?" Kyle pulls his Sentra outside of my second story apartment. We've been dating for a month and he already wants to see me more than I'm comfortable with. There's so much we don't know about each other still.

"Jen, I feel like you're keeping me out. I feel like I'm your Saturday boyfriend."

I cringe. I've heard these words before.

"Look, if you're seeing other people..." He trails off, bracing preemptively for my response.

What I should have said is yes. I've been in a six-year relationship with anorexia, a twenty-five-year soirée with obsessive compulsive disorder, researchers have paid to analyze samples of my blood to learn why I perform CPR on munchkins, and I'm five months out of inpatient treatment. What I should have said is that after I get out of his car, I will pretend I'm going inside for the night. But as soon as I see his taillights fade, I will go to the gym.

He knows I can't run anymore. I don't tell him it's because my bones are crumbling from years of starving myself. I don't tell him I'm in a relationship he can never compete with, that he should be far more afraid of this thing, that it would be better if I were fucking every frat boy within a one-mile radius. But I'm not. I'm sick. I'm five months out of a residential treatment center, the gym only just let me return with a doctor's note approving exercise, and I just gained five pounds that I hate.

God took running away. Fuck God. I hate God. Every time I've asked him for anything he's ignored me. I'm still mistaken for a runner, the sinewy calves and veins in my legs only attributable to two things. So when people ask me if I'm a runner, you're goddamn right I say yes.

The silence between us goes on a moment too long before I say, "No, I'm not seeing anyone else. I need to tell you something though." This is where I lose his respect, where he realizes I am a mess.

"Kyle, I used to have an eating disorder. I still have to manage it. It's pretty much under control though. But sometimes it makes it so I have to, like, work on myself and every now and then, I don't know, meals are hard."

He doesn't know I really like him. He doesn't know how many dinners I've delayed or substituted with garden salads just to be with him. He doesn't know that I should have listened to the voice warning me I wasn't ready, that my recovery was too precarious and I was starting to slip back into my old ways. He doesn't know how few people have made it through the filtration system, able to penetrate through the bond I have with my anorexia and engage me in an illicit affair right in front of its eyes.

"Kyle, I have OCD too."

I can tell by his response it will be a long time before he fully grasps what I mean. I don't acknowledge, even to myself, that I have misled him, blatantly lying to us both as if my eating disorder is a bygone tribulation.

He takes my hand. "I get it. I've dated girls with issues. There's nothing that could scare me off, Jen. I really like you. Maybe I shouldn't say this so soon, but I think I love you."

I hesitate. I don't love him back, not yet. Not until I get the sensation Angela has described, the infatuation with someone that makes her say things like, "I would gain twenty pounds for him" or "I would get pregnant for him." I don't feel that yet, so it must not be love. But I like him a lot, an awful lot.

"Jen, there's something I have to tell you too. I didn't want to scare you off either but last summer my brother died." He won't look at me, fixing his eyes on the sedan parked across the street, one wheel carelessly resting on the curb.

"Look, if that's too much for you I'll understand. I know we are new."

I wonder for a moment how anybody could be scared off by this. I want to be there for him. I'm ashamed that he's fought in two wars and buried a brother and I'm the one who needs treatment centers, stomach pumps, and dietitian appointments. I have no personal tragedy, no root cause for my self-created knot. I think about how strong this person is.

I don't tell him then, but at this moment I realize I could love him more than I have the right to. This person understands pain and his baggage is far heavier than mine. I suppress the wave of relief that washes over me.

Locked Up

"Fuck you. I'm not going anywhere. I don't give a fuck. I want to die. If you don't get the fuck out of here, I'm gonna fuck up both or you fucking fucks."

I'm in my last year of physical therapy school with two internships left until graduation. I haven't meant for it to be like this. It's the first time Kyle moved away, the first time we broke up. I'm handling it well.

Let me paint the scene. I've ripped down my blinds. There are ceramic shards from a broken lamp, innumerable vodka mini bottles, and half-eaten Klonopin pills scattered around my bedroom. Pop-Tart wrappers, milk jugs, an apple pie, and an ice cream cake line the kitchen counter. Vomit is splattered around the toilet bowl. Let's be honest, vomit is splattered in places even a ballistics expert couldn't explain. The ceiling, the tub, the curtains, the dog bowl... literally everywhere.

I try to sit up, but I'm too tired. Angela is here. Rachel is here. I don't know it at the time, but Rachel will never let me forget that it was her birthday.

"You're scaring Abby, Jen." Rachel knows my weakness. I look at my little spaniel, my best friend, and realize she's shaking. I can't allow myself to admit it's because of me.

"She's not scared. She just shakes sometimes," I slur.

"Jen, I called the police to do a wellness check. You can either come with us to the emergency room or the police can take you away on a mental hold." Rachel's calm, pragmatic voice grates in my ears.

"I'll lay out everybody up in this motherfucker," I say.

One of my many flaws is that my alter ego, Jen II, has an inflated sense of strength. She's confident she can beat up the strongest man and believes she wears an invisibility cloak to hide the most obscene eating disorder behaviors.

"I'm good, I'm good, I just tripped and broke a lamp. Fuck man, I don't give a fuck. Can you guys please go home?" I flop back on the ground, an angry limp noodle. Maybe if I close my eyes I will sober up. Nothing real can happen right now. I am in a dreamy haze, JennaLand. I'm dancing with my eating disorder. Angela and Rachel were not invited to the dance and they are trying to silence the orchestra. Nobody silences the orchestra when I'm dancing.

I'm convinced I've gotten fat. I don't know how much I've eaten, but at least $300 worth of food, not including the Steak 'n Shake on a separate credit card. I don't acknowledge the fact

I threw it all up. I never trust that I purged everything. These benders usually make me lose at least three pounds, sometimes more, but dieticians always quote an outdated, poorly conducted study where bulimics binged out of a vending machine and purged into a bucket. Their vomit was run through a calorimeter and it was determined that they absorbed half of what they'd eaten.

Shitty bulimics. Frauds. They weren't doing it right.

I am smarter. I risk a heart attack. I play with my potassium levels and wring out my myocardium, because I am much wiser. I kiss death, rinsing and purging, rinsing and purging for hours, then watch the room spin and patiently wait for my potassium and sodium to stabilize.

No less than three police officers arrive. An androgynous female cop pats me down. I don't recall if I was placed in handcuffs. There was a country song playing as we drove the less than five minutes to Aurora Detox Facility. And this is all I remember.

The next morning I wake up on a cot that smells like bleach. It reminds me of a gymnastics mat. There are no sheets and my shoes have been confiscated. I'm in state-issued sweatpants and my socks have grippers on the bottom, just like the postsurgical patients at my internship. The room is frigid, but a blanket of Klonopin still coats my brain.

A doctor is sitting beside my bed. I want to brush my teeth before I speak to him. Three days of bingeing and purging continuously, taking copious amounts of Klonopin, and chugging vodka are still clouding my comprehension that this is real.

"Do you know where you are?" I can tell he asks this question every day.

"Yes. Yes, sir." I cover my mouth with my hand, still self-conscious.

"What were you taking last night?"

"I was just having some problems... personal stuff."

"You tested positive for benzos and your blood alcohol level was three times the legal limit. We call that combination a mind eraser. Have you had any issues with substances in the past? Any hospitalizations?" He glances down at his clipboard.

I think back to five years ago, lying in the hospital, my stomach freshly pumped. I conjure the face of the smug young resident who told me that people who get their stomachs pumped once are more than three times as likely to have it done again. *Well, I didn't get my stomach pumped this time, asshole.*

"No sir, no issues in the past. I'm about to finish physical therapy school and it's been stressful."

It's true, I am about to finish PT school. Most of my time is spent in the back of the lecture hall calculating how many calories I have left for the day. I thought PT school would be a challenge, an endeavor worthy enough to replace my eating disorder, but it's just like undergrad and I'm no closer to becoming my own doctor. My main motivation for becoming a physical therapist was to learn the secret to hunchback prevention. I know the basics already, but I wanted to be the world's greatest expert and our program spent one day covering osteoporosis.

Soon after I take a nurse-supervised shower, the first meal is wheeled out to the common area. I haven't kept food all weekend, but I'm still high on Klonopin so I don't even bother to see what it is. Once the Klonopin flushes out of my system on my second day, my appetite returns with a vengeance. I can feel my ribs stick out of my shirt and I begin to panic. If I'm not released after three days, I'll starve. And I haven't eaten random food in front of strangers in... I can't even remember. I have no template for how that would occur. Rachel contacts my parents and the Aurora staff agree that if they bring me food, as long as it is sealed to rule out contraband, I can eat it.

A nurse's aide comes to my room and escorts me down a fluorescent hallway. Konkrete, a failed street rapper off his Risperidone, heckles me. "This girl never look at nobody. She just be lookin' at the wall."

I would love an excuse to take out my anger on Konkrete, even if he killed me in the process. But I resist. I walk into the visitor's room and my parents are on the other side of the glass.

"Honey, we brought some cottage cheese." My mom wears a horrified, desperate expression I wish I could forget. We are not the kind of family that needs to detox. My stomach rumbles at the sight of the carton. If all I eat for the rest of my life is cottage cheese, I'll die happy. Just something I can eat.

"Thank you," I say after a few too many seconds pass. I tell them about PT school and how I'm miserable. About how all

I can think about are bodies when I study cadavers all day and I need a break. My mom tears up. I know I'm disappointing her by dropping out. That's what it is, isn't it?

"Mom, I'm sorry. I have a plan though. I want to be a teacher like I wanted to my freshman year. I know it's not enough money, but it would help me keep my mind off my own issues. I want to help kids and make my life about that."

She's too choked up to speak for a few moments, and when she's finally able to, she whispers, "Your hair, honey. Your hair looks like it hasn't been brushed in days. You look so... terrible."

Bone Thug

The reason Kyle and I break up for the 117th time is not particularly important nor interesting. Suffice it to say it's over location. Over Spring Break I fly to see him in Virginia, where he has moved to pursue his dream job. I'm not in a good place in my recovery, which is a recurring theme. After dropping out of physical therapy school, I switched career trajectories and became a teacher at Chestnut Middle School. Education was my true passion before I switched paths to become an expert in my own spine.

I maintain a weight that is almost sufficient to control my bingeing and purging, and my thinking is more rational with the extra pounds. There's a threshold for my brain and it hovers around 93 pounds. I function as a normal, somewhat limited human being at this weight or above, but when I drop below it I plunge into a world of irrational rituals, panic around food, and erratic weekends spent bingeing and purging.

Maybe I don't wash my hands before lunch one day. Maybe I walk through an old woman's sneeze going into Walgreens. Or maybe a student licks his hand before turning in his paper. Whatever the reason, I have diarrhea. I'm not shy about it. In fact, I relish in giving my Work Mom, Klein, all the juicy details as we chat in the hallway between classes.

My bowel history includes an impacted colon and a doctor sticking his finger up my ass after two bottles of magnesium citrate fail me. Complications from constipation are so common in anorexia that in residential treatment all patients are required to take Miralax each morning.

So this diarrhea is a welcome change of pace. I am unbothered with the prospect of the food I put in my mouth being jetted out within an hour, nearly lifting me off the toilet seat like a geyser creating a reverse bidet.

What I choose to ignore is that the pound of weight I lose must be mostly brain tissue, because it takes me just over the edge to reveal my anxious, neurotic alter ego, Jen II. The one who latches on to benign ideas and chases them with the fervor of a starved dog. When I cross into this territory, I insist my neuroses are a result of terrible OCD and entirely unrelated to my eating disorder. I spend my time trying to clear my mind of obscure worries, which distracts me from eating disorder recovery in the process. This leads to further weight loss, and the vicious cycle continues.

Shortly after Kyle and I became official, Dr. Styles had given me several options for medication. With his guidance, I chose Brivina, a shot given four times a year. At the time it was relatively new and researchers had not yet discovered that it has one terrible side effect. After three months it wears off completely and puts users at risk of vertebral fractures, or in other words, spinal collapse. Hunchback. Had Dr. Styles or I known this, I would never have chosen this drug that I now can never discontinue. My osteoporosis diagnosis is the first real consequence I've suffered from anorexia. It took away running, and the idea of becoming a hunchback horrifies me to this day. I comfort myself by promising I will commit suicide, which is soothing for about ten seconds until I realize that I'm also terrified of death.

After a year on the potent medication my bone density improves dramatically, and it continues to improve with each shot. It never returns to normal, but I am no longer at an acute risk for fractures so long as I stay on treatment. To someone without OCD, this would be a relief. To me, it is a constant source of paranoia. Whenever I am struggling, it revolves around Brivina and my bones, the modern-day munchkins.

My memory of the visit to see Kyle is relatively foggy. When the plane lands in Reagan airport, the rotund man next to me jokingly says, "That was a crash landing!" I'm not amused. Kyle waits for me in baggage claim with a hug and a Pike Place coffee, but I spend the next two hours researching which airports have short runways that could cause a harsh landing.

I pull up case reports of every old woman who has ever broken a bone on an airplane and wonder if during touchdown I unwittingly became a hunchback.

Lil Snupe passes away and Kyle is unmoved, which deeply bothers me. We see the cherry blossoms, visit Mount Vernon, and drink at a bar named Spider Kelly's. But suddenly I worry that his sports car has a firm suspension, and I refuse to ride in it. Every seam on the George Washington Parkway feels like it's traveling up my spine, and I imagine my vertebrae collapsing like dominos as we drive. Kyle hopes that I will grow to love Virginia and consider moving in with him, but as I'm fond of reminding him, I will never leave Sanford. Standing in his kitchen, we agree that we have no future and the visit ends awkwardly.

Once I return to Sanford, concern about the safety of my current exercise routine overwhelms me. Almost three years of physical therapy school made me an expert in body mechanics, and I know about basic contraindications, but I need the reassurance of a professional. I don't find it suspicious that this becomes an urgent need as soon as I drop below the magic number, 93 pounds.

Over the years, I have become a regular on the National Osteoporosis Foundation forum boards. I'm mostly a wallflower, too nervous to post anything for fear that my words in black and white will jump off the screen and strangle me, crushing my spine in the process. But I enjoy reading about Windblown, a great grandmother trying strontium citrate. There's DXAGuru, a retired radiologist who will answer questions about bone density scans. And Scott, who received his diagnosis after years of Prednisone used to manage his Crohn's. And then there's me, J-bones, biting my nails in the privacy of my own home as I read horror stories that will later crawl into bed with me.

I need the expert of all experts. I need somebody to watch my form on every single exercise and pick it apart, critiquing it to tell me I'm going to be okay. Enter Sandra Leeks, the premier expert in body mechanics. She's my version of Elvis, Michael Jackson, or even Lil Scrappy. She's a local celebrity, a rock star that nobody but me and Windblown and Scott knows about. And she happens to live right across town.

Taking a break from my diarrhea, I make an appointment. I want to show her every exercise I've ever done so she can evaluate it. I ask Angela to take a few video clips of me at the gym. I spend an hour on the elliptical trying to perfect my form, and the whole next day at work I can hardly function as I rewatch the clips in my head and try to predict what Leeks will say. The anticipatory anxiety in the month before my appointment is a convenient excuse to miss meals, purge away my apprehension, and distract myself from the fact that my major issue, actually the reason I have osteoporosis in the first place, is my anorexia.

My first appointment is on Friday the 13th, which should have been a warning. I leave directly from work and drive to east Sanford, past St. Patrick's Catholic School where I used to have basketball tournaments, past the Walmart I wasn't allowed to visit after dark in high school, and into a charmingly dilapidated neighborhood where Leeks lives with her husband.

There are two steps leading up to the doorbell, and she greets me with a hug like we are old friends. I step inside of what appears to be an elaborate home gym. There are diagrams of spines, each vertebra labeled, on her wall. Beside the spines is a large poster of a teenage girl in a papasan chair curled up with a book. Her spine is in full flexion, and the menacing words stamped over her read **SLOUCHING TODAY WILL MAKE YOU SORRY TOMORROW**. There are anti-fatigue mats in the foyer and two standing computer stations with ergonomic keyboards, allowing Leeks and her husband to stare into monitors directly at eye level. Immediately to the right is a kitchen and living room straight out of a sitcom on TV Land, as if the Shrine to Spines never existed.

We begin immediately. She is long-winded, which exacerbates me. When I seek reassurance, my desperation for instant answers is insatiable. I want her to watch my clips from the gym. I need her to tell me that my form is perfect, that I'm doing just the right things, and that I must keep doing exactly what I'm doing. I want to be told that any fear in my mind is silly and I could never become a hunchback.

Then I want to leave and never see her again. If I even inadvertently see her face pop up on LinkedIn, if Facebook reminds me it's her birthday, if there is any event to trigger her memory at all, I will picture that girl in the papasan chair and see my life flash before my eyes. I'll see me hunched over in my kitchen, about to commit suicide in a way that is still to be determined.

"Before we get started, I want you to color a picture of the three layers of back muscles. These are the muscles you must keep strong. I want to be sure you understand all of them from superficial to deep."

I spent three years in physical therapy school to master everything there is to know about the back, and I'm annoyed at the elementary exercise.

Next she wants to know about my medical history, which seems like an irrelevant topic. I am semi-honest with her, because Leeks is all-knowing. I reveal everything but my eating disorder, using the term "ran too much in high school" as a euphemism. She examines my previous bone density reports, asks about family history, and shows no indication that she is nearing the end of her interrogation. The hour creeps by like I'm wading through sludge but is over much too soon.

No, Leeks. This is not what I want. I want to ask you questions. I want to be told my worries are irrational.

Her thorough approach confirms what I've known all along, that my bones are crumbling and I'm going to be a puddle of mayonnaise by the time I'm thirty. Finally, we get to my videos. I scribble smiley faces on my notepad to send my future self a smoke signal that Leeks is not telling me to stop working out. But she's also not meeting my reassurance criteria.

I swing too much when I do bicep curls. My back does not stay flat against the bench press pad. I rotate my pelvis when I do renaissance rows. I pull back with my biceps instead of my scapulae when executing a horizontal row.

To me this feedback is more difficult than being told I'm probably infertile, or that I will never get a period without hormone replacement therapy. That news hardly penetrated my brain, but Leeks' feedback wrecks me. The gym is the one place I escape to. I had to give up running and the idea that I could be further limited terrifies me. I can't let it happen again, not ever.

Leeks wants to see me again. She wants me to retry the exercises with her suggestions and meet back in a month. This month will feel like an eternity, and on top of that I'm still processing the break up with Kyle. My diarrhea is a consolation, but it doesn't soften the blow. In fact, I actually have to see a doctor, a strong-framed, serious man of around forty who tells me after prescribing the antidiarrheal, "Be careful. You don't have any weight to lose." I'm used to these warnings, but never too concerned. Doctors just want to make me fat. My priority is Leeks.

I spend the next month ordering tripods of all different sizes and angles so I can take as many videos as necessary for Leeks. I need her to see my new and improved form. I spend hours in the gym, but I wait until the middle of the night so nobody will see me film myself and think it is for vanity reasons. It is for Leeks reasons. My stomach is in knots for days before my appointment. To my delight, my follow-up with Leeks goes better than expected and my exercises gain the official Leeks Seal of Approval. She applauds my perfect form and emphasizes the importance of strength training. I can't wait to never see her again as I gather my things.

But as I walk down her steps, she calls after me, "I think you should check back in with me again in June. We can go over some other information."

Maybe if I weren't me, I would have said, "No, thank you." I would have kept my $100, having gleaned the wisdom I needed out of my first two sessions.

But I am me. She wants to see me back and now I am stuck in a terrible reassurance loop with Leeks, the 5'3" woman who carries a posture correction pillow everywhere, warns me not to sit down for longer than an hour at a time, and whispers in my ear every time I curl up on the couch with a good book.

Straight spine. Straight spine. Straight spine.

My saving grace is that I have not talked to her about bulimia or my eating disorder. We discuss every exercise I could ever perform, every bus I could ride, every bedroom maneuver. I leave no stone unturned, but I don't bring up this one taboo topic, which allows me to assume purging is still healthy.

Since becoming a teacher, I have tried to get a handle on the purging. I'm by no means recovered, but what used to be once or twice a week is now once every few months. I no longer misuse Klonopin, only taking it when I'm truly panicked. But on this particular afternoon, I don't want to think and I definitely do not want to feel.

Forget Kyle. I don't care about Kyle. I want Leeks to watch me do the chest press again. I want Leeks to show me her front squat form. I want to bury my emotions in Leeks. I'll never need Kyle again. I'm done being good, tired of avoiding old ways, sick of needing to do everything perfectly all the time. I've gone from one extreme to the other, from purging almost every day to living in fear of it, and I'm sick of walking on eggshells. I'm caught in the purgatory of being 40% recovered from an eating disorder.

I pull into a gas station to pick up a case of beer. A girl who looks to still be in high school approaches me.

"Excuse me, miss. I forgot my ID. Do you think you could buy me some beer? Here's a twenty. You can keep the change."

She's a baby, cornrows clinging to her scalp, long fake eyelashes batting at me convincingly. But I'm not going to risk my career to buy her beer.

"Can't help you there," I say, accidentally sounding like a teacher.

I put my case of Michelob Ultra on the floor of the passenger seat and crack open one bottle, dump it into a Styrofoam coffee cup, and scan the parking lot for cops. Halfway through my first, I realize there's not enough beer in the world to drown out the noise.

I walk back into the gas station. The young attendant looks at me suspiciously. He probably thinks I'm on this side of town to buy drugs. The absurdity of that. I buy an overpriced package of Tylenol PM and wash the pills down with beer. I crush up the other two with my teeth and let them dissolve under my tongue, the diphenhydramine reaching my bloodstream almost instantly. For good measure, I root through my purse and find one loose Klonopin. I hold it under my tongue until the residue shoots straight to my brain.

I ride through town, stopping the car only to pour another beer. I suppose I could get a DUI but I decide I just don't care. I don't want to think about Leeks. I don't want to think about Kyle or my spine or Rachel. Rachel insists that I'm relapsing. She's never believed in me.

I look at my ab muscles in the rearview mirror. This weight loss is suiting me well. All the muscle I've built over the years is popping through. Losing a few pounds has accentuated my figure. My muscles look round and full and there's not an ounce of fat over them. J. Cole is thumping through my stereo. *No Role Modelz*, indeed.

The novelty of driving around drunk grows old. The world doesn't look so pointless after the chemicals hit, and I change my plans for the evening. I'm usually regimented with my exercise. Fridays are cardio, a mixture of the elliptical and stair climber. Saturdays are back and biceps. Sundays are leg day. Tuesdays I squeeze my rectus abdominis until I feel as if every muscle fiber will tear off my ribs, but I manage to do so without once flexing my spine. And Thursdays are chest and triceps.

The routine is helpful for me to limit myself. Putting boundaries on how long I can exercise and how much cardio I do helps prevent a relapse into the compulsive exercise that introduced me to Kyle in the middle of the night. I set my watch timer and when it beeps, I leave the gym.

But today I'm a little bit drunk, a lot a bit buzzed, and in the most clear-cut way possible, in denial and out of fucks. I know there is no chance I can eat tonight. All I will do is read and read again my notes from Leeks. I'll fret over which exercises I need her to approve next. I'll check public records for the property she owns, court records for any medical malpractice claims, and online blogs to see if anyone has ever been led astray by her advice. Leeks is now a God, an omniscient entity, and anything that casts doubt on her credibility must be excavated. I put my trust in her entirely, but I'm at the mercy of what she says.

I'm not ready to go home to my eating disorder recovery convent. Not today. I'm thankful for the diarrhea. It showed me how great I look after I lose a couple pounds. Lately strangers stop me to compliment my bulging muscles, nickname me Mighty Mouse, mistake me for a gymnast. I've always had muscle, but losing the fat over them gives them an extra pop, doesn't it?

People with eating disorders don't get compliments on their bodies. Not if they are really sick. The only place I want to be to release all my pent-up aggression is the gym. But first I need to counteract all these chemicals. I'm not willing to wait hours to sober up, so I stop by a Daily's gas station. They really are nicer here.

I purchase four exorbitantly expensive white Monster Zero energy drinks. I snap my first can open as I return to my car and proceed to chug three in succession. The cold, fizzy bubbles rush down my throat, quenching my cotton mouth from the Klonopin and sleeping pills. I save the last one, the fourth one, to carry into the gym like a badass, ready to show off. I'm tough. I can't be fucked with. Nobody will know I sit at home fretting over what a 78-year-old posture Nazi will tell me. Nope, not me.

I wish I had cute workout clothes. All of my clothes are baggy. I'm too self-conscious. And even when I do find something that feels comfortable and looks good, I never wear it. I save it for a special occasion that will never come. Because they never come. Maybe I'll fix that soon. I'll give myself a makeover and buy some flashy new clothes to show off my biceps.

I'm ready to rebound and start over with anyone other than Kyle. Kyle and I are too intertwined, too codependent. I've been listening to relationship podcasts and taking online quizzes, and we are not a healthy couple. He knows too many things about the cogs and wheels inside my brain. There's too much opportunity for me to leak my darkness all over us both, spreading my dysfunction. I want a new, happy guy who won't see through my facade, who will never peek behind the curtain and see the destructive person that I am. I hate that Kyle knows what I will say before I can say it and sees every paranoid thought when he looks into my eyes. I have never been so open with anyone, and it has backfired. A sorrow shared is a sorrow doubled.

I clutch the fourth energy drink and strut into the gym, wrapping my ego around me like a blanket, or more accurately a curtain hiding my meltdown. I realize alcohol is wonderful fuel. I don't need food. Energy drinks are great. I can take Klonopin in moderation.

I float on denial and dopamine. I leave the gym hours later and decide it's time to throw caution to the wind, take every scratchy worry and propel it out of my body, and coast on the fumes of emptiness. My first stop is Moe's, followed by Cold Stone. I don't look at the prices and feel no guilt as I drive to the grocery store for more. I have plenty of money in my savings account.

I wake up the next morning to a scene reminiscent of my 72-hour hold in college. Splatter covers the toilet. Thankfully no broken lamps. I realize I left my wallet in my trunk, so I walk out to my car, still half awake. Unfortunately, I forgot to bring in the birthday cake milkshake from Cold Stone. The early morning sun is a kiln, permanently binding the vanilla, speckled film to the fabric. Despite this setback, I'm still riding high off of the release from the night before, and even this doesn't ruin my mood.

I cook a new breakfast. My recovery meal plan calls for a bowl of oatmeal and a cup of blueberry yogurt. But this morning, I choose a bowl of brussels sprouts instead. This way I can cut my calories for the day and fill my stomach. These are old habits, but they feel like old friends.

The wagon was stupid. I don't want anywhere near the wagon, because last time I was on the wagon it drove me to Sandra Leeks, who whispers in my ear every time I bend down to tie my shoe, pet my dog, or sit on my couch.

No forward flexion. Straight spine. Hip hinge. Proud chest.

Shut up. Shut up. Shut up.

As I wait for the brussels sprouts to steam, a sulfuric aroma filling the apartment, I download a dating app. It's like Amazon shopping, except instead of browsing for posture pillows, I'm searching for men. Swipe right if you like, swipe left if you don't.

I have a few criteria. Nobody over six feet and nobody over 200 pounds. I don't want to be crushed during sex. Nobody with a boat in their profile picture, threatening to fracture my spine on every wave. Sandra Leeks went on her brother's boat, but she stood the whole time to protect her spine. Boats are the school buses of the sea, and this restriction narrows the field considerably. *Sorry Sean*, I think as I look at the tall orthodontist with the toothy white smile, holding up a big mouth bass. *You are missing all three of my criteria.*

I go on a couple of dates with no connection. Coffee with Jeff from Singapore, who has ordered me a cup by the time I arrive. I would never drink coffee if I didn't witness it being poured. It might be poisoned with butter. And the fact that he ordered for me is an immediate turn-off. Any hope of chemistry is neutralized as my coffee grows cold.

But then I match with Jason. A year older than me, 5'8", 170 pounds. He is applying to med schools, loves to read and work out, and does not own a boat. He is the exact opposite of Kyle physically, yet somehow both men are my type. In his pictures, he wears oversized diamonds in his ears and dresses in solid-colored polos that are safely fashionable. His teeth sparkle against his dark Trinidadian complexion. I'm nervous to meet him, and I assume he'll be disappointed.

We meet outside of Royal Cinemas to see a Marvel movie that requires 3D glasses. I overlook his choice in movies and decide three hours of boredom is worth it if we form a connection. I have Leeks on my mind, so I'm careful not to twist too far in my seat as I talk to him. He breaks the "no talking in movies" rule, and between the explosions and flying dragon balls, our conversation flows easily. I'm diligent about using the bathroom every 45 minutes to an hour so my spine doesn't compress. But apparently he can't see my wheels turning, and he suggests we continue the date at a local brewery. Without the sound effects in the background, I notice he has a slight Trinidadian accent. I play Kyle's role this time.

"What kind of music do you like? I actually won tickets to a Kendrick Lamar concert last year."

"I like rap," he says. I'm excited to compare notes.

"Who's your favorite artist?" I pray he doesn't say Migos.

He hesitates too long. I can see his mind flipping through an empty Rolodex.

"Jay-Z," he says finally, but there's no confidence behind his words. "I like how Jay-Z... sings." And then he starts to laugh. "To be honest with you..." That's how he starts most of his sentences. It sounds annoying but it's charming.

He drinks surprisingly little, stopping at one rum and coke. My drink options are limited. There are no domestic bottles of beer, which makes it impossible to track my calories at the end of the night. Instead I order Diet Coke and vodka, but because I don't know how much alcohol each drink contains, I'll have to skip breakfast and lunch tomorrow. But it's worth it if I want a new life.

Midnight strikes and he walks me to my car. He kisses me goodnight, and the kiss lasts a long time. It's not the kind of kiss where he wants to come home with me. It's the kind of kiss that is just because. A Just Because Kiss.

On the drive home I reflect on what a nice night it was. Things don't have to be so complicated, and starting fresh with someone new has shown me that. Then I remember that when we met in front of the movie theater, Jason greeted me with a hug. He gave me a little squeeze at the end.

Jason is perfect. Perfect height, perfect weight, intelligent, kind, ambitious, loves basketball, doesn't own a boat. But maybe it's not going to work out. If we go on two dates a week for six months, that's 52 squeezes, and if it gets serious, which is the point of dating, he's going to squeeze me at an even higher frequency than twice a week. I'll become his personal rubber ducky.

Jen, no. Don't do this. Don't let your toxins leak onto Jason too.

But I can feel the mice in my head scurrying around, my old baggage still not able to fit into carry-on.

My screen lights up with a text from Jason. **Hey, I just wanted to let you know I had a really good time tonight. It's been a long time since I've clicked with somebody like that. Never laughed that hard on a first date.**

Maybe it was my drink straw impersonation of a walrus. Maybe it was my tale of a student shoving poop into my pencil sharpener during my first year of teaching. Whatever it was, we clicked. It's ridiculous to worry about a hug.

The typing bubbles are still going, and the anticipation is excruciating. Finally, my phone lights up again. **Would you want to hang out again? Maybe go to dinner sometime this week?**

I'm confident this time. Dinner doesn't scare me at all any more. Wherever he chooses to take me, I'll order lettuce. Jason is obviously attracted to my body, so he won't suspect I have an eating disorder. I'm much more nervous about the pre-dinner hug.

Dinner sounds great. Are you free Wednesday?

But that's not what I need to say. I want to start this relationship off with honesty, and I promise myself I'll ask him to stop hugging me. On Wednesday, we meet at a casual diner.

I order lettuce and sprinkle it with Splenda when he's not looking. I drizzle soy sauce over the leaves and he doesn't blink an eye.

"You're really into your macros, aren't you?" he asks, but there's no judgement. He has already felt my stomach, and my abs are a selling point for him. Everyone has always told me my eating disorder is a disease, but I've finally learned how to make it into a healthy lifestyle. I'm relieved that there has been no hug. It must have been a fluke, a first date squeeze. After several hours of talking about family, life goals, and previous relationships, he walks me to my car. To my horror, he leans in for a hug. I stop him and decide to disclose all of my issues right up front.

"Jason, I have osteoporosis." I try to look as casual as possible, as if my entire life does not revolve around avoiding a hunchback.

He takes it very well but looks confused as to why I'm telling him miscellaneous medical information. Then I continue.

"To manage it, I have to work out to keep my skeleton strong, and also watch my posture." I trail off. The next part is what I really need to say. "Oh, and one more thing I almost forgot. Strong hugs are a little bit risky. Do you think you could squeeze me a little bit less tightly when we hug?" I feel the heat crawl up my neck and nervous red blotches form on my chest. I know this is a bizarre conversation, but if I don't lay it out for him, I'll find an excuse to sabotage our fling before it starts.

The next few weeks, Jason and I go to places I've gone many times before, but it feels brand new. I feel brand new. But he's missing big chunks. He's starting to wonder why I never invite him over and why he's never spent the night. The reason for this, of course, is that I am not eating when we're together and I am losing control in private. I can't admit to myself that I have relapsed completely.

I cover my pain with shameless narcissism. I'm in love with my reflection for the first time in my life. I buy flashy new workout clothes. I get lots of compliments on my muscular, lean physique, which only adds to my delusion. I'm free from the three square meals of a treatment plan. Recovery is a cage of routine, and I'm not willing to live a dull life any more. It takes a few weeks for me to look at my bank account and realize what I'm doing is not sustainable. I'm struggling with an old problem, but it has escalated to new heights. Every night after my normal days with Jason, I binge and purge.

I try to control it by bingeing on safe foods that I won't purge. My vice is carrots. Most days I can't make it to noon without inhaling three to four pounds in my car, too famished to even wait until I get home. For larger meals, I close my eyes and pretend a bowl of pumpkin and Splenda is pumpkin pie. But most nights, I end up in drive-throughs and gas stations buying food to throw up all night. Chunks of hair fall out in the shower. I seldom sleep, and it surprises me how little this affects me. Rachel warns me I am on a bad path, and this is not flexibility. She urges me to return to inpatient before I lose all control.

Jason sees a tiny sliver of me, and he's drawn to it. He sees a gem in the middle of a forest, but I know if he flips me over, he'll find the maggots and worms and earwigs as they scurry away from the light.

I'm only concerned about purging because I have not demonstrated it for Leeks. I would never bring up purging to Leeks. It's never been something I've been able to control well, and I don't think a medical professional would advocate for purging being a safe activity, bones aside.

But my ribs start to throb from the muscles I use to force the food up. The cartilage that connects to my back becomes overused and inflamed. I fear that any back pain could be a vertebral fracture. A hunchback is even more terrifying now. I feel like I've finally found happiness, and having to kill myself and end a life so sweet is unacceptable.

I form a hypothesis. Maybe I'm only purging because I'm anxious about my spine. Purging hurts my ribs. My ribs aching triggers the fear that I've broken my spine. I purge to cope with that fear, and the cycle continues.

The only solution is to get an X-ray to make sure I have no fractures, and then I will stop purging and live happily ever after. If a doctor performs a morphometric analysis of my spine and confirms I have no fractures, I will stop purging and continue with my new flexible life. I'll return to the honeymoon stage of my relationship with Jason and find true freedom from my eating disorder.

I'm terrified of primary care physicians. I never want one person to know my entire medical history. Then they will know I am insane, and I want them to like me. So I keep them all separate and pretend to forget the names of certain specialists. I want each doctor to focus her attention on the exact reason I am seeing her. *Why does my gynecologist ask me about my eating? What does that have to do with my vagina? Why does my dentist ask what medications I take? Does he need to know this to clean my teeth?*

Doctor shopping and doctor avoidance are two sides of the same coin. Receiving health information is so stressful that I avoid medical care and neglect even routine check-ups. Until I don't. Then I seek out medical advice excessively, but only at urgent care centers where there is no doctor-patient relationship or continuity of care.

I choose CareClinic for my X-ray, but this time go to a new location so I don't run into the same staff that treated my diarrhea several months ago. To my disappointment, the very same doctor enters the exam room, the same wooden face. I hope he doesn't remember me. He probably sees ten cases of diarrhea a week, I convince myself.

I lie and say my back hurts. I do not care about my ribs. My ribs won't give me a hunchback. I want him to X-ray my spine, and he orders the test. After ten unbearable minutes spent envisioning life as a hunchback, he walks into the exam room and closes the door behind him. I bite the inside of my cheek until I taste pennies.

There's a somber look on his face that mismatches his words. "There are no fractures. Your back is fine."

The numbness of relief temporarily paralyzes me, a sensation almost identical to a nearly missed head-on collision. I get off the table and he asks me to sit back down.

"Lie back," he says, reclining the table. I'm bewildered. I only came here for an X-ray, no less, no more. He palpates my stomach, focusing his attention on the right upper quadrant. He pries my eyes open and examines the whites, looking unalarmed.

"Do you have a history of liver problems? Hepatitis?"

I'm caught off guard. I've done my share of chemical experimentation, mostly Klonopin and alcohol, but I also go weeks and sometimes months without a drop. Liver issues have never occurred to me. "The sclera of your eyes aren't yellow," he says, seeming pleased.

"Hold out your hands." I follow his instructions. I feel like my dog, anxiously waiting for a treat after I shake her paw. After a long silence, he blurts out the reason behind this impromptu examination.

"Why are you orange? Do you realize that you're orange?"

"I'm not orange. I don't think I'm orange. Am I orange?" I simultaneously argue with him and ask him. I look down at my hands and they are glowing. But they have been for weeks, and I've been so worried about my spine I haven't bothered to wonder why. He places his hands, palms up, next to mine. His flesh is tannish pink, but not orange. Next to him, I look fluorescent.

"I eat a lot of carrots. Could that be what it is?" I try to decide if I want to admit just how many.

"You would have to eat pounds of carrots every day for that to happen. Have you lost weight since I saw you for the diarrhea?" *Fuck, he remembers me.* "You need to get bloodwork."

I'm aware that bloodwork will send me into a tailspin of compulsive online sleuthing. I'm paranoid that if any value is out of range, my insurance company will take away Brivina. It doesn't make sense, but I'm at a weight where logic disappeared long ago. Still, maybe if we build a doctor-patient rapport in these three minutes, he'll order the bloodwork for me and I won't have to see another doctor.

I level with him. "I've been having some food issues. Things aren't great right now and I'm trying to turn it around." The corners of my mouth curl involuntarily into a smirk. I can't keep a straight face as I minimize things to this extent. "Can you order the blood tests for me?"

He looks me over one more time. It's a quick scan, but his eyes are transparent. I imagine he would wear the same expression if he saw a hamster on a motorcycle.

"You really need to see a doctor, Ms. Dixon. This is out of my area of expertise."

Toilet Tisha

I'm thankful for Jason. Being with him is a vacation from myself. My personal life and my relationship are now completely separate, and I assume this can continue indefinitely. My plans fall apart when he sends me a cryptic text.

We need to talk. This is the male version of "I'm fine."

What's up? I try not to get grease on my screen, but I'm mid-binge.

Are you seeing somebody else? You disappear every night.

We agree to sit down the next day and hash things out. We meet at McDonald's because their menu explicitly lists the calorie content of their coffee. Jason lays it out for me. "You've never introduced me to Angela even though she's your best friend. Your mom and dad came to town last weekend but you didn't even ask me to meet them. And I've never seen your place. I just feel like you're keeping me at arm's length."

I have an explanation for all three of Jason's concerns, but I can't tell him.

1.) Why hasn't Jason met Angela?

My relationship with Angela had soured. She could see through my quarter-life crisis. She knew I was relapsing behind the scenes and hated me for it. My body simultaneously disgusted and triggered her, and I won't know it for months, but she and Kyle were now texting buddies.

Kyle: **She's just a monkey jumping from one branch to another. Good luck to Jason.**

Angela: **She's a bony little boy. Her arms make me want to puke.**

Angela had been distant for months, and I could tell she had no interest in meeting Jason.

2.) Why hasn't Jason met my parents?

I hadn't introduced Jason to my parents because I was nervous enough to let them see me. Shortly after my 72-hour institutionalization, and not coincidentally, my parents moved to a retirement community off the coast of Florida. After years of strained relations, we mutually distanced from each other.

My mom's departure email was a long time coming. **We've decided to apply for a job transfer to another city or state. We will take Grammy with us. Even though it will be hard for her, we need to try to get some semblance of a life**

back, remove ourselves from your therapy, and try to get some peace and happiness back in our lives. Your recovery will be yours. Whether you binge, purge, or starve, it's all your problem. You now own it 100%. I know we will have a normal relationship one day and I look forward to that.

I never visited them. Staying in their condo and eating meals with them was not an experience any of us wanted to relive. So several weeks ago when they called to tell me they would be in town for the day, the last thing on my mind was introducing them to Jason.

I couldn't let them see that I was still active in my eating disorder. I ordered two silicone butt pads off of Amazon to put in my pants. I prayed the butt pads, combined with two heavily padded bras, would add at least ten pounds. Combined with horizontal stripes, I prayed I could keep up my facade.

My parents suggested a hike. It was a steaming hot afternoon in the middle of a southern July, and hiking four miles in jeans, silicon padded underwear, and two bras cooked me from the inside out. I told them I couldn't go to lunch because my friend ChaCha Henderson wanted to meet up for focaccia and duck soup, but we made plans to get coffee before they drove back to their new home. Dad picked me up in his Rav4. I was scared to ride with him.

What kind of suspension does a Rav4 have? Is it bumpy like a boat? What is the aspect ratio of the tires?

Suddenly I heard my mom shriek as my dad slammed on the brakes, almost rear ending the hatchback in front of us. My seatbelt tensed, preventing me from flying through the windshield and becoming a hunchback mid-air. There weren't enough butt pads in the world to cushion that fall.

My seatbelt relaxed and my dad turned back to me. "Sorry about that. I didn't expect that car to stop." I could see that even my mom was no longer panicked. Relief must have been the normal emotion, but for me the event would live on for hours.

I scoured the internet on my phone, searching for key phrases. **Whiplash from deceleration. Compression fracture from slamming on brakes. Car accident compression fracture.** My parents could see me visibly falling apart, scratching my neck and unsuccessfully attempting to regain composure. I desperately pushed my nose as if it were a button to restore my sanity, a telltale nervous tic. I decided that the only way to salvage the afternoon was to get an X-ray after my parents left.

As I gave my parents a gentle hug goodbye, my mom told me how proud they were. I'm great at my job, I have nice friends like ChaCha Henderson, and I regained my composure quickly after my brief panic attack. I had come a long way in her eyes, a far cry from the insane girl raving about extra fucking beans in the fucking spaghetti.

As I watched their car grow smaller, I got into mine and rushed to GoNow Doctors, another doc-in-the-box. I was jonesing for another full spinal X-ray. It had been such a relief last time, despite being told I was orange. I was chasing that same feeling this time.

In walked a short, tidy man with a goatee and a ring of brown hair around a friendly bald spot. I instantly recognized him as a regular at the gym. My quest to remain anonymous in the medical system was not going well.

"Now this is one of the hardest workers in the gym," he said to the nurse. "Did you hurt yourself running?"

I tried not to bristle at the comment as it pried up the corner of my scab, exposing an underlying wound almost a decade old. "Yeah, I'm having back pain. I have low bone density, so I wanted to make sure I don't have a fracture."

He happily ordered an X-ray of my thoracic spine that he read on his tablet right in front of me. "Looks fine to me. No fractures."

"No microfractures either?" I ask.

"Well, those wouldn't show up on an X-ray. You would need a CT scan for that, but that's a ton of radiation." I make a mental note. *Get CT scan later.*

"How is my lumbar spine?" I ask.

"We didn't X-ray that because you pointed to your upper back."

"Oh, it's my lower back too. Sorry if I wasn't clear. Can you take an X-ray of the lumbar too?"

I was put back in the lead vest to protect my inhospitable womb, and once again the report showed no fracture. I covered both reports in smiley faces so my future self would know that I am 100% not a hunchback.

So that was why Jason had not met my parents.

3.) Why hasn't Jason seen my apartment?

The day that I moved into my apartment, I didn't see it as a dump next to the highway. It was my first time without a roommate, and I was excited to begin a new life where I could control the temptations in the pantry.

Kyle came over to help me unpack and christen it. When he went to take a post-coital pee, he looked at my toilet. The toilet was the most important amenity to me. My apartment hunt had been exhaustive, and as the leasing agents droned on about granite countertops or thick walls, my focus was on how high the toilet came up on my shin. Did the rim reach the tibial plateau or was it too close to my ankle? A comfort height toilet was ideal, but I also saw the value in a lower toilet where I could hip-hinge to purge. When I had used Leeks' bathroom, I noticed she had a low toilet. But I didn't think Leeks purged either, so I was unsure if this mattered.

My new apartment checked every box for me. It was affordable. It was a short commute. And I liked the toilet. Then Kyle killed me with two words. "Midget toilet." He called my toilet a midget toilet. Still riding the high of our romp in the kitchen, he had no idea what he had done. His words were a splinter straight to the brain. I spent the rest of the evening online shopping for toilet seat elevators, which placated my anxiety enough to not move out a day after signing the lease.

Letting Jason into my space gave him free reign to say whatever he wanted about the height of my toilet. It made having him over completely out of the question.

I could tell Jason all of these things, explain myself point by point. But where would I even start? There is no way to catch him up in one conversation. But I have to give him something.

"Jason, there's a little bit more to me you don't know about."

"Yeah, you're hiding something. You take hours to return my texts and something is so shady. I'm quiet when I notice things, but it's not like I don't notice them."

"What do you mean?" I wonder if he's implying he has noticed I have a hunchback.

"Like that you only eat lettuce. All I've ever seen you eat is lettuce. I don't want to hurt your feelings, because you know I think you're pretty. But I think you would look better if you ate more."

This segues into what I think at the time is a frank conversation. I tell him I have an eating disorder and I tell him I'm struggling. I don't tell him about Leeks or that Rachel has given me one month to find a residential treatment center. I don't tell him that I'm addicted to X-rays and I spend my spare time driving to different gas stations to check my tire pressure. I don't tell him that I'm losing my grip. I don't tell him that I'm starting to lose interest in him now that he knows. He's no longer an escape from myself, and even though it will take a few weeks, the flame has already begun to burn out.

False Prophets

Around this time, I reach out for help. Not by being more honest with Rachel. Not by paying attention during the dietitian sessions she requires me to attend. Traditional therapy is for true eating disorders. Over the course of the summer, I have discovered that I never truly had an eating disorder. I'm just a fitness chick who counts macros, as they say in bodybuilding parlance. So I seek help from strangers on the internet who will better understand.

Tara Taylor is an internet dietitian, and I find her approach much more tolerable than my dietician's. She has a YouTube channel where she talks about binge eating in the fitness community, and how it's nothing to be ashamed of. Her words comfort me as I binge in the dark, blocking out the hum of the highway outside my window and the chime of unread texts piling up in my phone. I send her an email.

Hi Tara,

I love your channel and can relate to so much of what you talk about. I was a runner in the past and then got into weight training about seven years ago. I am 26 years old, 5'3", and have ranged from 85 to 105 pounds during this time. My current weight is close to 90 in the morning and I am the leanest I have ever been. While I enjoy the vascularity and visible abs, I am starting to binge and restrict. I felt I looked okay at 100, but now when I gain weight I don't sit well with the added pounds. I do feel that my legs have lost some muscle, which I don't love, but my abs and arms are so much more striking at lower weights. It's a real mind fuck!

I always make up for the calories I go over, so my binges never lead to weight gain. However, it is becoming an issue mentally. I could use some accountability with my diet and some advice about what I should do with meal plans. I kind of think I need to gain weight to be healthy but I need someone to hold me accountable. I know my BMI is low but I have a very small frame. Does my situation sound like something you could help with? Thanks so much!

Jen Dixon

P.S. I'm sure this goes without saying but I of course would like this email to just be between us :-)

In less than a day, she responds.

Hey Jen,

Your current weight is very low as you mentioned, and this concerns me for your health. Binges can place additional stress on your heart. Ethically I don't feel online coaching is the best fit, and I urge you to seek the help of a local dietician that could monitor you more closely.

I totally understand the mind fuck, but I think getting some blood tests and finding out how to get your health on track is the best thing for you moving forward. I wish you the best.

Tara

My email back to her acknowledges the severity of my circumstance. She has made an impact on me.

Thank you, Tara. You could have taken my money or ignored my email, but your response was a wake-up call that encouraged me to reach out and get some help. But thank you for taking the time to answer me. Means a lot.

And I do reach out again, but this time to Lars Peterson, a bodybuilder who makes "hormone clinic" recommendations and runs a supplement company. But this time I reveal slightly less information. I don't want to give him the wrong impression like I did with Tara.

Hi Lars,

I have a question. Some people in my life say I need to gain weight, but I prefer my body how it is now. Do you think I look underweight or gross?

Sincerely,

Lyn Nixon

I attach a picture of my abs. It's not a sexy picture, just a zoomed in shot of my six-pack abs covered in roadmap veins. He responds even faster than Tara did.

That's impressive as fuck! Keep it up!

The pathology of my behavior is normalized in my head. My days are spent teaching and consuming self-help content on how to stop bingeing, and my nights are spent binge eating and purging. But I finally reach my proverbial rock bottom. So I think.

Soon after Lars gives me the green light to keep purging, I feel a sharp pain in my belly button. I hope it's a fluke, but as I reverse gulp, using every ounce of abdominal strength I have, the pain explodes. My hand moves down to my lower stomach and I feel a lump next to my navel. I turn to Google. **Hernia. Umbilical hernia.** Horrific pictures pop up of men with tumor-like bulges poking out of their stomachs, new mothers with mesh reinforcements to hold in their abdominal contents, and intestines spilling over belts. Just my luck. I've lived in fear of my intestines spilling out for nearly a decade, and it doesn't happen through a hunchback.

Nothing gets me to the doctor faster than fear of living with a permanently distended stomach, so I stop mid-purge, pause famous bodybuilder Rich Piana's *What I Eat in a Day*, grab my keys, and rush to the ER. After I check in, I have a few moments to think about my life choices. I'm about to suffer a real consequence for my behavior. Sitting there alone in the emergency room, I realize I have to change or my future will include many more ER visits. But I can't get rid of the voice.

You just ate so much food. You didn't finish purging. You still have Cheetos in your stomach, ready to be absorbed and turn you into a blob of fat. Nobody has ever eaten as much as you did today. You will gain thirty pounds overnight.

This is the last time. I will never purge again, but I can't let my last purge be incomplete. I finish dumping my abdominal contents into the ER toilet and pray my name isn't called before I finish.

Intake is embarrassing. My voice cracks as I explain that I injured my stomach by forcing myself to throw up. A nurse draws my blood and informs me that my potassium is dangerously low. I'm annoyed at the distraction. I am not concerned about electrolytes or heart health, which bear no relation to a beach ball stomach or hunchback. The doctor orders a CT scan, and to my relief the bulge in my stomach was actually massive quantities of vegetables clogging up my colon.

There are feces throughout the entire length of the colon, reads my CT scan interpretation. This is my unceremonious diagnosis. Severe constipation.

Relieved I won't need mesh reinforcement to hold in my intestines or any surgery that will cut into my six-pack, I decide now is my opportunity to get just one more X-ray. After this, I'll stop purging once and for all. They X-ray my thoracic spine. No fracture.

I am reborn. This is my fresh start. My rock bottom.

I walk through my front door, press play so I can see what Rich Piana eats for lunch, and immediately resume bingeing and purging. I'll start over tomorrow.

Tomorrow comes and nothing changes. I realize it's time. I've spent too many nights losing myself in bodybuilding blogs and pretending what I'm doing is the same thing. I am not a fitness chick. I am vomiting up my food. I am going to die if I don't get help and I need to be in an inpatient facility. Rachel was right. I can't do this alone. But first, I need to do some deep soul searching. Treatment is full of uncertainty and fear of the unknown. I center all of my anxiety onto a big white van.

Check In

Inpatient treatment is like boot camp for people with eating disorders. I imagine for everyone else, it would feel more like a resort. Chefs use the highest quality ingredients, and were it not for the table of weeping residents begging not to eat it, the food would be classified as fine dining.

Before eating, residents pass a laminated card around the table. On one side there is an anxiety scale. One is **Total Relaxation** and 10 is **Panic Attack**. Most of us report somewhere in the ballpark of 9.9 or 10. Next, we report our level of hunger from 1 to 10. Most of us wouldn't dare go above a 5 for fear that the CAs will mention we are hungry in the weekly staff meeting. This is where decisions are made about who needs more calories added to their meal plan.

The residents are from all walks of life, from the bubbly bulimic sorority girl to the woman who lived on top of a Circle

K for two years. During each of my three stints in this facility, I grow close with the other women. The CAs are easy to talk to, and they seem more like friends until we sit down at the dinner table. Sometimes it does feel like a spa. But most of the time, being watched as I use the bathroom, having blood drawn each morning, and accumulating demerits for unfinished meals make it feel more like Alcatraz.

I meet with a therapist twice a week, a nurse twice a day, a dietician three times a week, and a medical doctor as needed. I attend a psychodrama class where I embody a wolf and re-enact my birth. I receive a printout of my brainwaves during biofeedback. I sit awkwardly in group therapy sessions and try to list all the states from memory, hoping nobody calls on me to share. The only part of treatment that sucks is the treatment part; the lack of exercise privileges; the daily blood draws and weigh-ins; the stadiometer (and the constant temptation to measure my height); and for me, the big white van. And the food, of course.

If therapists are the Gods of treatment, dieticians are Satans. It's not their fault; they are doing their jobs. But if dietitians in inpatient eating disorder facilities want to be popular, they will be sorely disappointed.

Overweight dietitians can't be trusted. They try to trick us into becoming fat like them. But even worse are thin dieticians. They are traitors with evil plans to sabotage us through weight gain shakes so they can take pleasure in making us fatter than them. They hide their own issues behind desks covered with plastic mashed potato mounds and other patronizing portion-size models that belong in a nursery.

My first visit to the food farm was disappointing, but it did cure my addiction to exercise. I would later blame my own immaturity and re-admit myself to the same facility, convinced that getting older would allow me to finally tackle all of my issues and possibly uncover some deep chamber of my soul that causes me to self-implode.

The second time, I decided I wanted to learn to eat without a food scale. I chose to go to the same treatment center because I knew what to expect. Like many anorexics, I hate change. I couldn't eyeball normal portion sizes after years of using a digital food scale as a crutch. I was also purging all the time, but my goal was to cut ties with the food scale. To my horror, Maravilla wanted to treat my entire eating disorder, not just the part I wanted to get rid of. I was categorized as more severe than my first visit and denied almost all privileges. Activities such as walking, compulsive standing, and gym visits were entirely banned.

But the most offensive aspect was that my dietician required me to drink a weight gain shake three times a day. I was not here to gain weight. They did not share my vision. As the days went by the shakes grew bigger and bigger. (In reality the shakes stayed the same size, but the cups they were served in varied. This bothered me a great deal.)

"You're playing tricks. You're trying to fatten me up. I'm not here to gain weight. I just want to intuitively eat." I ended up sabotaging the visit in hopes they would kick me out.

My first text to Kyle after I finally earned an hour of phone time read: **Got caught sneaking almonds in my pocket today. Not held in high regard here. Fuck my life.**

But my third stint will be different. I'm older, I have a career, and I really really really want to stop purging.

Looking back, I can see that I made the same mistake all three times. I never went seeking recovery. I wanted to stop compulsions around food. I wanted to learn new skills. But I never surrendered. Surrender would have been going to recover from my eating disorder no matter what that meant, even if it meant gaining a lot of weight.

If I had semi-voluntarily gone to treatment twice, why am I so vehemently avoiding it this third time?

Rachel and I went round and round for months. It's not the food and it's not fear of weight gain. At least this is what I tell myself. I could lose any weight they forced me to gain, and it would be worth it if I learned to stop purging. But I channel all of my apprehension onto the big white van Maravilla uses for transportation. I picture it driving down the bumpy Tucson roads and see my spine collapsing. Under no circumstance do I want to be a recovered hunchback.

I don't think the facility in Arizona was particularly well run. There were girls purging in the house plants and sneaking out in the middle of the night to run to the gym. Different practitioners gossiped about each other in front of patients. My therapists often canceled or rescheduled my sessions, leaving me with lots of free time to gaze at the ceiling. Or in my case, become the MacGyver of exercise. My belt became my own personal Bowflex. I anchored it around the grab bar in the bathroom to do inverted rows. The toilet became my air squat platform. And my dresser became my pull up bar, with the added excitement of wondering if it would tip over and squish me under its weight. In hindsight, I could have tried harder.

But I choose the same treatment center the third time primarily because I've already ridden in their van, and I'd rather have the devil I know. My logic is that if I rode in the van twice already in my life, it is probably safe to do so a third time without consulting Leeks. I spend hours online analyzing Chevy E350 suspension, dampening, and spring rate. I ignore Rachel when she tells me I'm using the van as a distraction, that I'm once again letting my OCD get all the attention. I buy an ungodly number of Leeks-approved pillows to try to cushion any bumps. Finally, after exhaustive research, I book a flight to Tucson.

***

I'm sitting in Ann's office. Ann is my dietician, and she has called me in to review my meal plan adjustments after I failed to gain weight in my sixth week. But I have one thing on my mind, and that is getting exercise privileges. I can't even go on walks yet. I'm going stir crazy as I feel myself morph into the mashed potatoes model on her desk.

"Jen, you aren't healthy enough to exercise yet. Your body is in a very fragile state, and it could be dangerous."

Fragile. Fragile .Fragile.

The word burrows into my consciousness. *What does she mean that I'm "FRAGILE?!?!" Is she saying that my bones are fragile? Is she telling me that exercise is dangerous?* I already went through the whole process of getting my exercise cleared with Leeks. But she just called me fragile.

"What do you mean by fragile?" I need her to take it back.

She looks back at me with a frosty stare and I notice the nasolabial fold accentuated by her low weight. *Hypocrite.*

"You're seeking reassurance right now, Jen. We need to focus on increasing your meal plan. That's the purpose of this session."

Why are we talking about weight gain shakes right now? She just called me fragile. How do I know that my bones are okay if she's telling me I'm fragile? I'm not even anorexic. I'm a bodybuilder who can't gain weight.

I look at the veins running down my arms and think about Frank, the sultan of the gym. Even Frank told me I was too thin. *How can he think I'm underweight when my biceps bulge and I have veins all over my abs? I am the picture of health and strength. Why am I sitting in this cushy eating disorder clinic when I don't even have an eating disorder?*

Jen II takes the reins. "I don't even have a fucking eating disorder. Why the fuck am I here? I don't have a fucking eating disorder. I have terrible OCD and nobody can help me, and I'm tired of rotting in this place. I have no feelings to get to the bottom of. I'm leaving. I want to leave. Get me out of here." The words come pouring out, a faucet that can no longer be turned off.

"Jen, you told us you would try to leave. You asked us on your first day to not let you run this time. You came here to create a new life. Look at this letter you wrote yourself."

She opens my file and hands me a piece of notebook paper covered in messy scrawling. It's full of the naive optimism of the first day of treatment, before the shakes and van rides and sitting with feelings.

"What did you mean when you said I was fragile? What did you mean when you said it wasn't safe for me to exercise? All of my workouts are cleared. Leeks cleared everything." I'm in a thought loop and a simple letter isn't enough to pull me out of it.

I can tell she's done with me and the look on her face tells me everything I need to know. I don't sound reasonable. All of my fears make sense to me but I don't sound reasonable. I walk across the dusty parking lot, past the van, and back into resident lodging. The gravel gives a satisfying crunch under my feet. The smell of fresh basil and garlic surges into my nostrils, and I see all the other girls chopping up spices for a cooking lesson. Krista is still in her wheelchair. Her short hair is getting scraggly and her veiny arms look out of place hanging beside a protruding stomach. The research is conclusive. When an anorexic is refed, the fat is first stored around her vital organs. Her stomach. I can never let that happen to me. Plus, how will I know the belly is from refeeding? What if it's from a hunchback?

I picture the space between my ribs and hips shrinking and shrinking and my intestines bulging out. I run my hand up and down my stomach, feeling for every abdominal muscle. Every fiber of my being wants to go into the bathroom and make sure that the abs are still there. If they disappear, how will I know they'll come back? I can't eat if I don't have abs. That's what these people don't understand. I'm trying to feed myself, and every shake they pour down my throat will starve me later. I imagine what will have to happen when I get home, how many shakes I will have to burn off.

I'll have to get all of my exercise cleared again by Leeks, which will inevitably make me relapse. There is no world where I will accept a body that is imperfect. It's not just about weight anymore. Those were the simple days. Now it's about proportions and a straight spine. Every time I try to explain this, I'm accused of being in denial.

Ann must have called my therapist and told her I threatened to leave. Claudia comes in on a Sunday to persuade me to stay. I strategically dress in navy Hollister sweatpants and a pink Nike Dri-FIT shirt. I'm not dressed like someone with an eating disorder. I like Claudia and she's a good therapist, so it's difficult for me to disappoint her. She urges me to listen to the person I was on my first day, back when I wrote that letter.

"Jen, can you reread your letter to me? Read it out loud. The part about how your eating disorder will manifest as fears about bones and hunchbacks. You can't see it right now, but that is what is happening. The hunchback fear is just like the munchkins."

I'm calm now. I don't need anything from these people. I know that I will get no reassurance about the word "fragile." It rattles around in my brain.

Fragile. Fragile. Fragile.

The only way to deal with my distress is to discredit Ann, make any word that escapes her lips meaningless. She isn't much older than me, ten years at the most. She clearly doesn't follow her own plans considering she's emaciated under those floppy sun hats and flowy Bohemian outfits. Ann knows nothing. I don't need reassurance. I need to go home.

How could I be so stupid? This is the third time I've come to this place, and I've left every single time. I look out the window of the nurse's office at the other residents. There's Megan, who is having the time of her life here. She's still young enough to change. Krista is the one who dropped down to 50 pounds. Her feet swelled up so badly she couldn't walk for weeks. She was on a feeding tube for almost six months, and even she's doing better than me. Recovery isn't for me because I don't have an issue, and that is honestly how I feel.

I don't want to go through life being weak like those other girls, talking about my feelings in some cushy residential treatment center in Arizona. I won't binge and purge anymore.

I promise I will never do it again, because now that I've gotten all of those X-rays, I won't bend from the waist again. That was the whole problem to begin with, and I have every motivation not to put myself in that situation anymore. I have stood on death's door now, and I don't need to sit and process feelings for three more months.

I go back to my room and flop down on my twin bed. My roommate, Emily, fiddles with a Rubik's cube with no strategy in mind.

"What's the deal, kiddo?" Emily is my Rehab Mom. She has four kids close in age to me, and though I feel like I'm too old to change, she still considers me young. She's battled anorexia for thirty years, and she finally took out a second mortgage to invest in herself and stay here. "You don't want to end up like me," she has told me on my hardest days.

"I'm going home," I say. "This isn't for me. It's just not clicking."

"Well, you've been talking about going home for days. Maybe it's the right call. Everyone needs something different." She looks up from her Rubik's cube.

I'm surprised she doesn't give me the cliché answer, that I need to stick it out. It further confirms that I'm doing the right thing.

"Yeah," I reply. "I'm not going back to my old ways anymore. The past couple of months have been enough for me to realize I need to recover, and I just want to go back to my life and do things differently."

"I totally understand," she says.

At dinner, I'm surprisingly calm as they bring out my shake because I know I can leave tomorrow. An Uber arrives for me the next morning, and my first stop is Safeway. In treatment, eating large quantities of vegetables is considered an eating disorder behavior. But it's not for me. I just love vegetables.

I did have to drink a weight gain shake this morning, so one pound of carrots should be plenty for lunch. Other shoppers stare at me as I wheel two suitcases down the aisles, gazing at the overwhelming selection after weeks of having all of my choices made for me. I buy a bag of carrots and find a table outside the store. Eating in public will be a breeze compared to eating in front of CAs.

As I take my first bite, I realize that after weeks of eating real food, a pound of carrots for lunch is repulsive. *How did I ever eat four pounds a day?* I feel nauseous, throw the carrots away, and catch another Uber to the Tucson airport.

Starting Over

I don't remember much about the plane ride home other than emailing both of my bosses and telling them I'd be back on Monday. I have the whole weekend to regroup and get organized. The last thing I did before I left for rehab was box up my old apartment. During my layover in Charlotte, I call the movers so I can be in my new, fresh-start apartment as soon as I arrive home. It's the biggest place I've ever lived, a plush complex with residents who wear scrubs and walk poodles and hang seasonal flags. A new apartment will help me start a new life.

I also call Kyle. Jason and I broke things off shortly before my departure, and I realized in treatment that my heart remained with Kyle. I used every single phone pass to call him, and we decided to give it another try. But this time he's moving back to Sanford and we're getting married. There's no engagement ring, but it's understood that this is the end goal.

After the movers finish the heavy lifting, I'm left alone to bask in my new universe. I take in the beautiful fireplace and inhale the aroma of freshly shampooed carpet. The hearth creates a warm, inviting ambiance. This is a place I will bake sugar cookies and decorate with pictures of the memories I make. Me drinking margaritas with new friends and throwing the bouquet at my wedding. This is not the sort of apartment someone has an eating disorder in, and though the toilet is a perfect height, that's irrelevant now. I will never purge again.

I wake up the next morning and I am immediately overwhelmed. I don't know where to begin and I don't have any food to eat for breakfast. It's football season in Sanford, and school spirit is in the air. At the store, everyone is dressed in blue and gold as they pick up burgers to grill at tailgates. The default question the cashiers ask, knowing full well the answer, is "Do you know what time kickoff is?" I'm intimidated by the wide selection of food choices. I've become institutionalized from weeks of having all of my dietary decisions made for me.

I'm not yet at my target weight, but I do plan on getting there. Factoring in the weight gain shakes and all of the oil they cooked with in treatment, even if I overeat, there's no way I will get fat compared to what Maravilla fed me.

I was cheating in treatment. The almonds I would shove in my pockets, the water I would chug under the covers to create the illusion of weight gain, the air squats I would do while pretending to poop, all of those things added up. I don't know if I fooled them but I certainly fooled myself.

I carry the groceries upstairs and take out a bunch of bananas, slightly green to give me some time. I've never bought bananas because they are one of the higher calorie fruits. There are so many signs that I'm doing exactly what I need to in order to recover. I unpack the perishables and behold the sight of a full refrigerator.

I feel a pang of guilt as beautiful fall air streams in from my balcony. It's a gorgeous day and I have nobody to call, no friends, and even now all I care about is my next meal. The glowing green numbers on my microwave read: **10:17**, an hour before it's acceptable to eat. I can't sit and watch the clock all day. It's crisp and sunny, almost obnoxiously lovely outside. But I can't go for a long hike if I have to eat lunch in the middle of it.

All I need to do is eat all 1,800 calories I now allow myself. I can eat them all right now. Then I'll go to San Marco and take a leisurely ten mile hike. I never would've been allowed to do that at Maravilla. It doesn't matter that I'm alone. I have freedom, and soon Kyle will be here all the time. This is just a difficult phase, but soon my life will be better. I'll go to the gas station and get a Monster Zero, call Angela, unpack all of my things, and embrace this upscale apartment.

I watch my hand reach into a bag of Veggie Straws, satisfyingly crunchy as they congeal in the spaces of my molars. I take another giant handful. This is no big deal... but I throw the bag away as a precaution. I don't have a garbage can yet, so I put it in a lonely trash bag lying in the middle of the kitchen. Maybe I should leave to go to San Marco, just to be on the safe side. I know that I won't purge, and I've never had that security before. I trust myself 100%. I look at Abby sitting in the foyer, her humanlike eyebrows drooping. She looks bored. Am I boring? Why is food still all I care about? I'm hungry. I've been hungry for over a decade and I can finally eat without purging. Fuck it.

If I cram a bag of cookies in my mouth, will I keep it? For almost a decade, I have been sure I can immediately un-eat anything I don't deem acceptable. Suddenly overeating is just overeating. I take the bag of Veggie Straws out of the trash. Before my brain has a chance to catch up, as if someone else is plunging their hand time after time into the family-size bag, it's empty. I rip the bag open and lick every crease, every morsel of oil that has pooled along the tin lining, a habit that tends to develop when every calorie is calculated.

I feel uncomfortable, but it's alright because after this I won't have to worry about food. I'll fast and wake up tomorrow morning, back on track. Rachel hates it when I say those words, but she doesn't understand that I must have a clean slate to function. My eating moves quickly now. A box of Nilla Wafers- gone. I record on a piece of computer paper to make it feel organized. This is not out of control.

I drop a glass of soda. I'll pick it up later. There are a few small flecks of blood on my shin now, shrapnel from the glass. I'll wipe it away later. I don't care.

My body is perplexed. My binges are tens of thousands of calories when I purge. What will happen now? I'm 93 pounds, up four pounds after treatment. I know I need to get up to 100, but not like this. Slow and controlled, not like this. Surely my binges won't continue to be as enormous as they used to be. I only have so much space in my stomach.

I look at my pantry filled with food. It's stocked because I assumed I wouldn't struggle to keep food in the house anymore. I had my epiphany in inpatient and changed everything around me.

I continue to down cartons and bags of miscellaneous foods. I eye a box of Fig Newtons. I don't want to eat an entire tray so I douse it in soap and throw it away. Having a sudden change of heart, I fish it out and eat the bars that only have a little soap. Clean eating.

A two-day detox fast sounds alluring. I'll just take some sleeping pills after this and sleep through it. I can't take Klonopin. Not yet. I still have to go hiking. Get to go hiking. I want to hike.

My head throbs. I won't purge. This is just part of the process. My stomach feels like it's going to explode and I've never had to deal with that feeling. Not since I was 18, that dark year I've villainized for nearly a decade. That chubby little 99-pound failed anorexic alcoholic that I became, lying in the hospital after getting my stomach pumped, over-dramatizing everything. Stupid little twit. Now I see that my issues aren't that severe. I am in control and I'm not that weak little girl anymore. Two months ago, I would have already purged several times. I would feel empty and tired by now. Purging is no longer an option, but I feel too sick to move. I wonder if my stomach will burst and they'll find me dead, bags of Veggie Straws and Nilla Wafers filling my peritoneal cavity. How will the coroner explain the soap residue?

My mind flits to a song on the radio. *Unsteady* by X Ambassadors. I set my phone on the ironing board and watch the music video over and over. I look at the broken glass in the kitchen, at the blood flecks on my sock, at the plush new apartment, already tainted with me. Not with my eating disorder, but with me. My toxic essence. I'm too full to lie flat so I just lie on my side and try to breathe in and out. I wanted to gain weight, but not like this.

I open my laptop. **How many calories can you absorb at one time?** Some bodybuilders on YouTube challenge themselves to eat 10,000 calories. Cheat days. Was this a cheat day? I know I should take a Klonopin. I can't binge if I'm asleep. But I also can't build muscle. I need to go to the gym and put these calories to work. I need to have the willpower to stay awake and not binge.

I waddle to my car and drive down Franklin Avenue. I look at all the happy people. A little girl in an Eagles jumpsuit waving pom-poms on her dad's shoulders. Drunk college girls laughing and flirting with the baby-faced frat boys. I've been that girl. I couldn't quite keep up, and maybe a few 5150s and inpatient admissions should have clued me in to that.

I wonder if Angela is having fun right now. I want back in her life. I want her to know I've changed. I can change. I have changed. The old me wouldn't have resisted purging, but the new me did. I shoot her a text, knowing it won't be returned anytime soon. My optimism turns to anger and I'm too full to move, so I drive.

I'm fat. I starved my whole life to be fat and alone. I'm addicted to food, and I'm not like other anorexics. I won't recover because I'll keep bingeing.

To think, a week ago I was screaming at people about one shake. I just voluntarily dumped 4,000 calories into my body. The irony. Should I have stayed in treatment? Never left against medical advice? I can't entertain that thought.

I drive to Hillington, a stereotypical small town on the outskirts of Sanford. I need to gas up my car, so I walk into the service station and look at the drinks in the walk-in coolers. I'm too full to drink anything at all, but I'm parched from too much sodium. I eye the shelves full of bland energy bars, overpriced jerky, and pickled abominations. I glance at my watch. How could it only be 2 p.m.?

I wonder when all of the toxins and food bulk will be out of my system. The excess carbohydrates are pushing their way into my veins and I look like a snowman. Thin stick arms and chiseled legs pop out of a torso so stuffed with food it hurts to inhale. My six well-defined abdominal muscles are bulging, poking obscenely out of an inflated stomach. I have tortoise shell abs just like the failed bodybuilders with steroid guts. I hope mine goes away.

I ask Safari. **Can you permanently stretch your stomach out?** I fall down rabbit hole after rabbit hole of forums. Competitive eaters can train their stomachs to expand. Pregnant women can get diastasis recti, the repulsive separation that allows their lower abdominals to pooch out irreversibly. An hour goes by, me hunched in the parking lot filling my brain with information I never wanted to know.

I hear Leeks whisper in my ears. I shouldn't be sitting so long. It's bad for my spine. I'm doing everything wrong already. It's too late to change. I hate my life. I look at the front of the service station and I hate it. I hate my life and I want to die. I hate Kyle for leaving in the first place. I don't want to marry that fucker. He should be here. My mom should care. She gave up on me. Rachel is proud of me. She thinks I'm different. I want to be, but I'm not. I'm a fraud, an imposter. I think about family day at Maravilla. Nobody would bother to come to mine. My parents didn't even call. I was a lost cause the second they saw me behind that glass, a ward of the state for 72 hours. Fuck them.

I think of the video to *Unsteady*. A vulnerable, shaking alcoholic with his whole family worried about him in the somewhat valiant portrayal of addiction. He's a victim of his brain chemistry and traumatic memories. But I'll forever be considered a vain, superficial anorexic. And post-2010, I also picked up the Thin Privilege Badge of Honor. Somehow a physical manifestation of my suffering makes me lucky. My anger at the world turns inward. I'm a twit and nobody is around because I'm a burden who has worn out my welcome.

I unbuckle my seatbelt and walk back into the Shell. I grab a cereal bar off the shelf, Cinnamon Toast Crunch infused with dried milk. If I write down the calories I can figure out the math later. I'll save the wrappers so I can cross-reference and be certain. I shove my money across the counter and the bar is gone before I reach my car. I walk back in, avoiding eye contact with the attendant. Pop-Tarts would be the worst. I slept in a tree for Pop-Tarts. They have 420 calories in a pack. If I ate five packs, that's 2,100 calories. I would have to add 1.3 days to my fast.

I just need to get this urge out of my system. This is the last day of my life that I will ever binge so I'd better make it count. The cashier gives me a curious look and says, "Somebody was hungry." I look back at him indignantly. He has no idea. I've been hungry since I was twelve and I never want there to be an empty corner of my stomach again. I grab the bag, and before I drive away 2,100 more calories are gone. I stop by the grocery store on the way home and the rest is a blur. I eat 7,360 more calories on top of the 4,000 from that morning.

I wonder if I'll die. If I had just stuck to 4,000 calories and eaten tomorrow, I would be so much better off right now. Now I can't eat until Tuesday. What have I done? I have to go back to work, and the puffy face and inflated stomach are not my real body. I'm still sick, even with this most recent setback. I am still well under 100 pounds, but I step on the scale before bed and my 93-pound body has ballooned up to 110.6 pounds in twelve short hours. Now it's a game. How long will it take for all of that water and food inside of me to clear, and what will my frame look like when it does?

I wake up the next day and feel like I have a horrible case of the flu. My skin is hot and painful to the touch and there's a body-shaped imprint of sweat on my sheets. Both sides of my lower back throb and I can hardly lift my head. My feet are too swollen to fit into shoes and I realize that hiking San Marco is not an option.

Before I even attempt to get out of bed, I fumble for my phone. In a rush, I search: **Causes of lower back pain, paraspinal muscles**. Could intra-abdominal pressure from yesterday's binge put pressure on my spine as well? How ironic would it be if I got a hunchback from not purging instead of purging?

I can't allow this thought to cross my mind. Nobody has ever gotten a fracture from overeating. Obese people get lumbar lordosis, not kyphosis. I remember all the lower back pain patients at my internships in PT school, wanting massages or spinal manipulation when their real issue was that they were carrying around a forty-pound adipose baby.

I type: **Obesity rate in the United States** into the search bar and am immediately comforted. If two-thirds of American adults are putting their spines at risk of fracture, more of them would have hunchbacks. Being fat is fixable. Being a hunchback is not.

My phone rings. Kyle. I hate him. I resent him so much for not being here. I can still hear his voice. "We are going to get married. This is going to happen, Jen." Kyle has a confident air that makes it impossible to doubt him.

Shawn Murphy is going to find him a job in Sanford and I need to stay composed until he gets here. Once he's here there will be stability. Right now my life is in the middle of a transition and I need to be patient.

Looking back, I wish I had seen that the only common thread in every one of my experiences was me. The vulnerable alcoholic in the *Unsteady* video is a fictional character. I didn't want to look at what was really happening and I couldn't face the truth that I left treatment too early, unable to accept that I had fallen for my denial and believed it was about my spine.

After managing to find clothes that don't cling to my bloat, I lie flat on the floor. This burden is too heavy to lift. The only way to cope is to share it like a funny story, so when my sister calls I give her the comical version of events. We turn everything into a joke. But instead of the usual banter, she interrupts me, and in one of the most earnest moments of our relationship, she tells me, "That really sucks, Jen. I'm really sorry."

The empathy makes me feel worse. It further solidifies that I'm not a guru on YouTube doing an eating challenge. I'm not a bodybuilder. I have an eating disorder and I binged. And for a moment I want to talk to Kyle. I want to tell him I'm struggling without getting irrationally upset at him. It isn't his job to fix me and I know it. He didn't sign up for this.

I think back to my days singing in an embarrassingly amateur youth choir at the church down the street. My family had never gone to church, but my sister was banging the drummer, so to speak, so we both joined. We sang pop songs and dissected the lyrics, searching, perhaps reaching, for ways to tie them back to Jesus.

I gave the introduction for *Lean on Me*. I was eleven years old and a bit of a ham. I loved public speaking, and though I lacked musical talent, I was eager to introduce the song. The message of *Lean on Me*, I told the congregation, is that a joy shared is a joy halved while a sorrow shared is a sorrow doubled. As soon as the words left my mouth, I heard the hee-hees and muffled giggles of my choirmates. I had gotten it backwards. But maybe I hadn't. Maybe I was the only one who got it right. When I let my struggles spill over and share them with other people, my mess becomes their mess and it smears like a stain. The one thing I can handle today is my food. I am the expert, the master of manipulating my weight, and that is beautiful.

I shuffle into the gym later that afternoon and realize I don't care. What's the point of working out? That burns maybe 200 calories when I'm in a surplus of 9,560. Lifting weights will just rev up my appetite, and I'm so bloated that no amount of muscle will show for a very long time.

For a moment, my rational brain gives me a bird's eye view and I hover above the petri dish that has become my life. I supposedly left Maravilla so I could continue to exercise and not have to see Leeks again. It had nothing to do with calories. I was totally fine with gaining weight, not scared at all. So why would I not work out just because it hardly burns any calories? Could I be in denial? I don't think so. I'm just going through some changes.

Nobody at work will know that I put on all of this weight in the last 48 hours. They'll probably assume that I'm cured now, as if inpatient is a course of antibiotics. All the weight sits under the surface of my skin. I think back to a picture of myself when I was a chubby little sixth grader playing Shakespeare in a school play. I have on a Renaissance hat and a black wig, and a pen-drawn beard fails to hide my moonface. I look in the mirror and that is exactly how I look.

You look like a dumbass Shakespeare, I tell myself, and laugh hysterically. But it isn't funny. I just need it to be.

My embarrassment about my weight gain should be a sign that I'm missing the point. I'm still too proud to surrender and allow myself to eat. I don't want the world to see I've given in to my carnal desires and grown weak.

I'm Back

My first day back at work, a fellow teacher who I am not particularly close with is waiting for me in my classroom with a hug. I try not to focus on it. I try to focus on how sweet she is, how surprised I am that she cares. A hug can't give me a hunchback. My classroom neighbor pops her head in to welcome me back. "Look what the cat dragged in," I preemptively say before she has an opportunity to ask me how I am. The one person I want to check on me is Principal Lutz.

I've read enough armchair psychology to know that how I feel about her is not normal. Maybe it is related to the tumultuous relationship I have with my own mom. Sure, she has slipped into the early-onset dementia that's been leaking into her cerebrum for years. But she was never strong. She was never a role model. I love her immensely, but my feelings toward her are conflicted. I spent my entire life seeking her approval, but also looking down on her domestic, vanilla existence. She never had a career. She made scrapbooks, joined the PTA, and shampooed the carpets once a week.

Lutz is a power-woman, not concerned with pleasantries or even being liked. She's the new Coach Maddox, existing somewhere in a parallel universe to Rachel. The Rachel to my work life. Maybe I'm getting too old to need a strong female to place on a pedestal, emulate, rely on to show me how to be. But somehow I still do it.

I want Lutz to like me now that she knows this piece to my life, this dark corridor of my mind. I had to tell her I was going to treatment, and though I dreaded the conversation for weeks, she was understanding. She told me about her own battle with cancer and how health comes first. I thought the chat, alone in my classroom before the first bell, brought us closer.

I don't want anybody else to ask me how I am because I don't want to share with them. They ask and I answer, "Doing fine," in an awkward tone meant to end the conversation. I will never tell them I have an eating disorder. They have no wisdom for me. Sharing a piece of myself with Parrish or Hartman, as sweet as they are, serves no purpose. I want Lutz to ask me. She will have wisdom. I want her to be concerned and to know I'm a fighter. I don't know why, I just do.

I love my students as they trickle into the room. I look at their innocent faces. The behavior issues that turned my world upside down two years ago are now the lowest of low on my priority list. They hated their long-term sub and I secretly revel in that fact. They try to share horror stories about her and I half-heartedly tell them not to speak ill of other adults. But in the back of my mind, I remember that I am good for something other than an eating disorder. I'm a great teacher who can get the most apathetic students to understand and actually care about learning. And that means the world. At least it did until my eating disorder ruined that too.

This year I'm much more laid back. I wear T-shirts under my jacket. The days of trying to act like a hard-ass, like a stickler who rules with an iron fist, those days are over. I have a rapport with my students, but they know I'll lay the hammer down when necessary. The classroom, my colleagues, the culture- it keeps me going and reminds me that my eating disorder is only one part of me. I missed this. I wasn't happy being a useless, inert invalid, shut away in some hotel for weirdos in Tucson.

The end of my first day back arrives and I've now been 24 hours without food. My body is still bloated, but my stomach screams for nourishment and I love it. It hurts worse than any thought. I'm still at a surplus of 7,760 calories, but if I don't eat again tomorrow I can be back on track by the weekend.

The dismissal bell rings and a stray thought hits me. Nails me actually, right in the corpus callosum, the fibrous band that holds the two halves of my brain together. I envision it burrowing so deeply that my brain splits right in half. Fucking thoughts like this are like ticks. I can pull them out but the head stays in my body, embedded in my brain tissue.

Dr. Styles has retired. *Where will I get my Brivina from now? What if another doctor won't prescribe it for me?* My bones will crumble and I will be a hunchback. I don't want to have to kill myself. I'm not suicidal. Getting a hunchback, the idea of having to do that to myself, end it and become dust... I can't let that happen. I can't be negligent and force my own hand, force my own self-imposed demise. *What if I was too scared to even do it and allowed myself to exist in this world, all hunched over, intestines protruding as people whispered about how tragic I was?* I have to secure the Brivina injection for January and I have to do it now.

PubMed. It's a work computer but I don't give a shit. Nobody would even understand what I'm looking up. I type in: **vertebral fracture cascade** and the terrifying results populate, pages of studies about the dangers of stopping Brivina. Not only will it stop making my bones stronger, it will also put me at risk for vertebral collapse. The very worst side effect imaginable.

I think back to a stormy afternoon in 2012 after my third consecutive bone density scan showed bone deterioration. "It's time to get on medication. You don't have any bone left to spare," Dr. Styles told me. I pressed the mute button on my phone so he couldn't hear my sniffles. He gave me two options for treatment.

Brivina or Norteo. Brivina or Norteo. I laid down on my bedroom floor, laptop open, and researched my two options.

The self-assigned project lasted days. J-bones asked for help from Windblown and Scott. I registered as a doctor on Medscape and paid to break through paywalls. Kyle sat beside me rubbing my legs and hoping for more. We fucked on my bedroom floor right in the middle of me reading a post from DXAGuru.

If we hadn't fucked, would I have chosen Norteo? Brivina was probably a mistake, but I really had no options. How is a 23-year-old supposed to pick between a drug she will need every three months to avoid withdrawal fractures or a drug she can't stay on indefinitely because it may cause cancer? It doesn't matter anymore. I'm stuck on Brivina for life and I have to find a doctor to prescribe it. I don't care if it means no pregnancies. I would gladly pay that price to save my spine.

It's only October and I've been home for three days. I can't handle this. Food will make it go away and I'll become more stressed about eating, and then all I'll have to worry about is managing my calories. The Brivina worries will be put in perspective. Food is the pathway to instant clarity. I don't even want to be on track with my food because then I'll have other problems I have to deal with. I want to fuck my food up so badly that it's the biggest problem in my life and ten times more stressful than any phobia about hunchbacks.

My contract stipulates that I stay on campus until 3:30, but I rush out the door, averting eye contact with any administrators. I clutch my invisibility cloak and rush through the sea of minivans and helicopter moms. I drive to the dollar store around the corner, grab a box of sugar-free shortbread cookies, and inhale all 24 before I bother to put my credit card back in my wallet. Then I drive to YoLites, an ice cream parlor that specializes in air-infused diet ice cream. What is 200 calories of ice cream compared to all the calories in those cookies? I calculate in my head that I have eaten over 200 grams of fat in the cookies alone.

I console myself by hoping that the cookies will be like a laxative, coating my digestive system with slippery globs of fat so I can rid myself of all the pollution I'm stuffed with. The wonderful thing about the hyperfocus on steroids known as OCD is I can justify any situation, bending steel bars with ease to make them fit my anorexia's will.

Did I just consume another two days' worth of food? Yes. Is this the second gigantic binge I've had since I got home from treatment? Yes. But I have also eaten 200 grams of fat and maybe that will help unblock me. Maybe that will actually have a reverse effect and my metabolism will speed up. I know it's bullshit, but I need a grain of hope to hang on to.

As the cashier rings up my ice cream, my eyes land on a case of high-fiber, sugar-free brownies for $4 a piece. I buy four of them, along with another eight-ounce cup of ice cream. I let the ice cream and brownies warm up on my dashboard as I find a YouTube video about resting metabolic rate. I want to convince myself that my overeating will counterintuitively lead to a leaner physique. I run out of patience waiting for my sins to defrost and cram them violently down my throat. Almost

$20 of food is gone in five painful gulps and a brain freeze. I immediately go back in and buy the exact same order all over again, lying to the cashier that it's for the next day. This cover story will become even less credible when I return tomorrow and repeat the entire process over again.

This time I have the patience to find a good video. Rich Piana. He's up to 330 pounds. The human growth hormone he injects, combined with eight meals a day, has allowed him to gain a pound a day. I need to watch somebody who is not fat scarf down food along with me. As he shovels chicken into his mouth, he preaches to me about eating big to get big and how muscles need nutrition.

I walk into the gym with my stomach protruding under a baggy T-shirt, bursting with ice cream. I see the same gym regulars, bench pressing and rowing and running and lunging, probably not thinking about Leeks. I go to the lockers to store my wallet and see a large, muscular frame with dark hair. Frank. He reminds me of a shark, but the gym is his ocean. His taut facial skin makes him appear twenty years younger and slightly like Frankenstein.

"Where have you been?" he asks. His stocky training partner scrolls through his phone, uninterested in Frank's distraction.

"I got sick," I say cryptically. I want him to put two and two together, but I don't want to say it outright. I want him to know that piece to me, to know that he was right and I'm sorry for shutting him down when he warned me about my heart last year. I regret lying, telling him right to his face what he knew was a lie. I was sick then, but I'm different now. I'm not afraid to gain weight.

I just stuffed my gut with thousands of calories and I'm here. I'm not hiding because I'm not wrapped up in how I look any more. I know everyone saw me shrivel down to nothing, waste away to sinew and bone, a selfish bony little boy walking around with a pencil neck thinking I looked buff. The vanity, the embarrassment. I have so much to make up for, so much to prove to everyone.

I hope Angela and her fiancé Jeff are upstairs. I have never seen Jeff on any equipment except the bench press, his stocky frame patiently counting out reps of five. Rest, talk, repeat. But he doesn't like me. He has OCD and he doesn't let it get so bad. I'm doing a bad job managing mine. At least I was. Now he'll see I've changed, and he'll tell Angela I'm worthy and I should be invited to pool days again. If anything, the way I look right now, bloated and nourished in the worst of ways, will help me mend things with Angela.

I want my best friend back, my other half. The friend who told me that if one day I'm a hunchback, and if I can't get better and I go insane, I can live in her basement. I can still feel her arms around me as she wiped away my tears, sitting on my bedroom floor as I processed the results of my first bone density scan.

"It's okay, Jen. I promise, if it all falls apart and you become a hunchback you can be my creature, and we'll watch *Real World* and *Celebrity Rehab* every night. I'll chain you up and call you Creature, and I'll feed you through a slot under the door." Angela knew how to make me laugh through the darkest of times, and I need that back.

I walk up the second flight of stairs and look at the rows of benches filled with people I care about. I don't know them. What's the point? I can't go to lunch. I can't do anything. But of all places in my life, I fit in here. No food is served here. Whatever I choose to be my soundtrack rushes through my ears and validates whatever emotion I feel as I exorcise the demons in my mind.

I take comfort in familiar faces. There's Frank. He's the most important because he has wisdom. But there's also Chris, a lanky Jamaican guy with a dragon tattoo, friends with Kyle originally. Years ago in the lobby as noise poured in from the woos and claps of the ecstatic Zumba posse, Chris introduced me to his boyfriend. But I couldn't hear for certain if he said "boyfriend" or not, and now it's too late to ask.

Then there's Short Chris, not to be confused with Chris, my sister's middle school boyfriend. She towered over him back then. Except now he's not Short Chris, the drummer kid in band. He's Chris, a pharmacy professor. He's Chris, who asked me last summer, "Do you take calcium? Do you ever take a day off?" It almost ruined our rapport, and had he not dated my sister for nearly a year, it would have.

"Do I have a hunchback or something?" I asked him, briefly dropping the agreeable smile I paint on to mask the anger and fear and stress. No, now I'm dead serious.

"No, not at all," he answered quickly, awkwardly, uncomfortably.

Minutes later, as I rested between sets of Leeks-approved squats, he came over. "Look, I'm sorry. I shouldn't have asked medical stuff. That was over the line. I just meant you're really lean, but it wasn't my place."

"No problem," I replied, the smile mask now fully back in place. Short Chris didn't know he stole my lunch that day, the ever-elusive promise to eat foiled by his attempt to help. I forgave him, and guilt washes over me now as I realize I'd made him uncomfortable. My stain, my mess had somehow seeped into Short Chris' morning workout. My neuroses were not his fault, and now that I'm recovered he will see that I've won, I've beaten this disease, and I'm no longer that girl. I don't want his friendship, not outside of the gym. But I want him to know I'm not a loser, that I haven't lost to what he knows is lurking underneath the surface.

None of these people know me, nor do I let them. But these relationships are close in a distant way. If I saw them outside of this setting I'd have to stop and talk, and I'd want to. Like the time I saw Chris at the store, his cart full of Budweiser and cold cuts for a Super Bowl party. The Doo Dahs vs. The Lee Loos as I recall... I don't follow football.

That day I realized he is not in a calorie prison. Maybe he goes home after the gym every night and his boyfriend prepares dinner. Gazpacho with pretzel sticks. That's a normal meal, right? Maybe he and his boyfriend take turns getting up to feed their baby. Maybe he's not even gay. I'll never know. But today is not about Chris or Short Chris. It's about Angela.

I need Angela and Jeff to be upstairs. I hate what I see in the mirror, but I'm proud that I don't look sick. I don't wear the scarlet A, the Anorexic Cloak that works better than any DEET to repel everyone who sees it scorched into my skin.

Now that she's going to see me get sloppy, all of the competition will be over. I thought so many years ago that I wanted to win, I wanted to be skinnier than her. I hated her bicep vein, her oblique muscles jutting out of her bikini. I hated her tapeworm, hated that she stayed skinny even after she did what I've never been able to and recovered for a guy. But I am skinnier than her so I won. I won a game that has no prize and I lost my best friend, and control of my life.

Thank God those days are over. I'll lose the sloppy weight, drop back down to 93 pounds, and gain in a slow, controlled manner. But first I want everyone to see that I'm better, that I'm different. Different from my old self, different from the fragile anorexics in the movies.

Angela and Jeff are not upstairs. I scan the benches and turn right to the pulley stations. Is that Angela on the lat pulldown, sleek ponytail swinging as she substitutes scapulohumeral rhythm for a slight arch of the spine? Poor form for her, death sentence for me. But alas, the girl with the careless spine is a doppelganger, a tease. I go downstairs. Nowhere. They aren't here. I'm back in town, I look healthy, and they aren't here.

Nobody else talks to me. I never take out my headphones. Chris and Short Chris and Frank are not my friends. They are acquaintances. People smile hello, but that is not a friend. This is the one place I thought so many years ago I could find like-minded companions. If I could be a bodybuilder or date a bodybuilder, my behavior around food would be accepted. It would be normal, desirable even, to weigh every morsel on a food scale. But even in this subculture I'm too rigid. My cheat days are binges done in private, inhaling Perky Jerky and Quark in my car. Their cheat days are margarita glasses and T-bone steaks at Outback. They train together, but I won't do anything Leeks hasn't approved of. I'm bigger now, but I'm still alone.

The realization stings until I remember I have one friend that will always be with me, and that is food. I stared death in the face last summer. I'm me and I'm living my own way. I have created my own world now, just like what I had with anorexia. Now I have food games, but they are healthier, and before long I'll be normal enough to have friends, get married, and even visit my parents.

For a moment I wonder- am I finished being suicidal? Am I really done with all of this or do I want everyone to see me heavier because I know it's temporary? The Klonopin days are over. The haze, the chaos, I'm too old for all that. But am I done with everything yet?

I look in the mirror and I hardly recognize myself. Inside I'm broken. I've never felt so sick. The Brivina anxiety seeps back in.

Find a doctor. Don't be a hunchback. Don't be negligent, find twenty doctors.

After all that food, the head of the tick is still embedded. I leave the gym, doomed to research doctors all night. I don't bother to pick up a weight. It won't make a dent in the surplus I've created. It won't make me accepted. It doesn't matter.

After my shower, I send Kyle selfies as I lie on my carpet in a black spaghetti strap shirt, hair all around my head. I send them as a joke, the punchline being my swollen face.

Hot, he texts back.

I'm uncomfortable with the response. I'm not hot right now, I'm fat. I want him to laugh with me, laugh at this imposter who is renting my body. I pinch together the fat on my stomach to resemble a mouth and FaceTime him.

"Hi Kyle, I'm Fatty McFatterson." *If my problems were about an eating disorder, I wouldn't be able to do that.* He doesn't laugh.

"Babe, you look awesome. Please don't lose weight. This looks so much better. I wanna bang you so bad right now."

Banging is the furthest thing from my mind. I'm annoyed at the suggestion, but also glad I'm bangable. Better than the alternative. He talks about his boss. I wonder how long his boss will be his boss. When will he link up with Shawn Murphy in Sanford? I picture Shawn Murphy offering him a job that will finally unite us.

My Hood

A few weeks later, Kyle takes me to stay at his childhood home in the Keys for Thanksgiving. His mom, Lisa, lives in a small, fancy house. The floors are covered in artisan rugs she acquired in her travels around the world. She's a slender, blonde woman, and she's undeniably attractive in the most natural of ways. Her skin shows her age, and years in the sun have formed lines around her eyes and down her cheeks. The deep crevices demand respect and insist she get credit for years of earthly experience. Yet somehow it doesn't detract from her beauty.

She's thin, almost frail, and I wonder what she thinks of me. I don't have to wonder too hard. I know that she doesn't care for me, not because of any direct interaction, but because of her perception that I'm going to hurt Kyle. I know she thinks I'm a project for Kyle, a fixer-upper. That Kyle is trying to save me because he couldn't save his brother. I wonder sometimes if she's right.

She gives me a tour of the house and I'm surprised at her warmth. Kyle has been evasive enough for me to ascertain that his mom is slow to approve of any girl he dates, but Kyle and I have an especially tumultuous past. At this point we have been together six years and broken up countless times. We always patch it up and reunite stronger than ever, allowing a callus to form around whatever the breaking point had been. But what is water under the bridge to us, material for inside jokes and silly rhymes, is not so amusing to the people around us. They tend, without exception, to pick sides.

Micah and Jasper used to belong to Kyle's brother, but they are Lisa's now by default. They're littermates, but you would never know it. Jasper is black, short-haired, and massive, while Micah resembles a fawn. Kyle and I have brought our dogs, Molly and Abby, and a pecking order has yet to be established. All seven of us walk down Patterson Avenue, past the small animal hospital where Lisa worked for twenty years and the nursery school Kyle and his brother Joe attended, a tiny building within walking distance.

Lisa tells me about her travels and I listen attentively, trying to erase her preconceptions that I am a trainwreck sucking her son into my toxic orbit. Sometimes I resent Kyle, because if it weren't for his recounting everything through his own biased lens, his inability to see things from any perspective other than his own, maybe it wouldn't alienate me from his friends and family. Maybe if he told them about his jealousy, his searching through my emails, the New Year's Eve we broke up and he laid on my bed, dead weight, and refused to leave. Maybe they'd see that my toxic orbit is our toxic orbit, that we are two toxic beings stuck in a magnetic spiral, attached by emotional scar tissue too thick to sever.

When we get back to Lisa's house, Kyle jumps in the shower and I bring my suitcase into our room, what used to be Joe's room. I think about what Kyle told me, how it's only in movies that the paramedics clean up. I look for any splatter, any flecks of blood left on the wall. The room has probably been repainted. I imagine Joe, drunk, upset, service weapon in his mouth. The impulsiveness of it, the carelessness. And I understand it, and that terrifies me. I imagine the sweat on his headphones, still wet from his workout that morning.

Kyle comes back to the room, beads of water still on his chest. I want him to admit it, to own his own shit for once instead of taking it out on strangers in traffic, on perceived slights from the Verizon salesman, on the people he'll never see again. I want him to admit that's why we hardly see his dad and younger half-brother, why he shows at best indifference toward Vincent. That he doesn't want a new puppy, a shiny new toy brother blessed with the two-parent family and club soccer team that he and Joe were denied.

Lisa has cooked a rich pasta boopity bop. I assume Kyle has told her in advance that I won't be partaking, and I already sheepishly stocked her fridge with enough food to sustain me for the week. I sit with them and overcompensate, oversell my passion for teaching, over-smile and over-nod. I wonder if it works.

Lisa retreats to her bedroom to unwind for the night. It's almost 10 p.m., and the acid in my empty stomach begins to burn. My appetite has been managed all day with countless Monster Zeros, McDonald's coffees, sugar-free Sparkling Ices, a bag of lettuce at Exit 66... but at a certain point, hunger cannot be suppressed. At some hour, some moment, some heartbeat, it breaks through the caffeine, the sedatives, the alcohol, and the exercise, and it begins to grumble. The lower you go in weight, the longer you engage in these torturous food games, the louder it screams.

I have the food I need. Two veggie burgers, one bowl of oatmeal, an entire bag of steamed broccoli covered in calorie-free syrup, and a cup of diet cocoa. I'm eager. Eager isn't strong enough- I'm desperate.

I find Rich Piana on YouTube. He's doing a challenge to inject more HGH and less IGF-1. But there's drama between him and Bostin Lloyd. He slept with Bostin's girlfriend, and a nude photo leaked showing that Bostin has a small penis, barely eclipsing his shrunken balls from years of juicing.

I need to watch smut when I eat, now more than ever. The pettier, the trashier, the better. I have the attention span of a lizard, fight or flight mode activated, and smut is what works just long enough for me to relax my throat and let the calories reach my stomach, lets me absorb the food and not bring it back up. Plus, Rich Piana is always changing experiments on himself, like a self-contained human laboratory. It reminds me that everything I'm going through is normal, that everyone is doing bizarre experiments with their bodies and I am okay.

I'm aware this is not my home and I feel guilty for bringing my own food, like a presumptuous and intrusive villain. I'm the wretched girlfriend in the Lifetime movie, about to be replaced with the agreeable southern peach played by Reese Witherspoon. I feel guilty for eating, ashamed for using the refrigerator, embarrassed of a body that takes up so much space in her home.

But I don't know what else to do. Rachel told me it wasn't a choice. If I wanted to travel, I had to commit to planned meals. I couldn't risk a starvation-induced outburst or starve for a week. I couldn't risk my recovery. She made me repeat it over and over again. "I do not risk my recovery. I do not restrict. I will die."

I send her pictures of the food and updates about Rich Piana. It's how she knows that I'm still following my meal plan, that I haven't thrown all of the food away and started researching vans or X-rays.

I arrange the broccoli on my plate, ready to hear what Bostin will say back to Rich Piana. I drizzle the calorie-free syrup over the leafy florets, then dust them with salt. I'm almost ready to escape into a world where my stomach isn't empty, where I've managed my food, where I can sleep. Suddenly I hear footsteps and pray I turn around and see Abby, or Molly, or even Kyle. I can eat in front of Kyle.

My stomach sinks and my heart races as I see Lisa come out of her room and pull up a chair next to me. She wants to bond. She's let her guard down and suspended judgement. Clearly I am not the same girl Kyle described, and she likes me. She tells me about birds in Portugal, tying trackers to their legs, conservation, and other words that hit my ears and fall back onto the table, a disorganized collection of verbs and nouns. Syrup on broccoli. She's going to see. *Does the broccoli smell bad? Is there any in my teeth?* She's incredibly sweet and I'm touched at her effort to connect with me.

My stomach is in knots. *Do I save the food for later?* I can't do that. A meal is a perfect window of time, a mini-era that I can't get back. *Do I eat and try to talk to her at the same time?* I take a bite but I'm still chewing when it's my turn to respond. I swallow the floret, unchewed, and it travels down to join a pile of bricks in my stomach, a knotted rope of anxiety and terror.

Rachel texts me, trying to pull me back to the meal, not knowing why my updates have stopped. **What's going on? Are you still eating?** I'm supposed to send an update every six minutes during meals, a sign of life in the form of a random fact about celebrities and rappers.

It would have been easier if Lisa had walked in on Kyle and me. It would've been less private, less intimate. I'm here for a week, and building a relationship with Lisa is more important than a plate of broccoli. I look at her delicate earrings and her wiry arms and it occurs to me that she might be thinner than me. She might be thinner than me but has spent her life traveling to exotic lands, helping birds and petting lions. I wonder what she thinks of me, if she thinks I'm a malingerer, a fraud.

She didn't see how sick I got. She is seeing the aftermath, the pudgy, stocky, thick aftermath, 99 pounds of failure after years of starvation. The imposter. I am 99 pounds of salt and fiber, fat and subcutaneous fluid. I look healthy, but I still put syrup on broccoli and need Rich Piana to scream at me, steroidy veins bulging, just to eat. I made this disorder up. I need to be like Lisa, thin but with no eating disorder.

I let the broccoli grow cold and send Rachel a cryptic text: **I did fine tonight. Just didn't need the protocol.** The protocol is the strict regimen I must follow each day, and proof that I stick to a meal through pictures of food and celebrity updates is Requirement #1.

I get into bed with Kyle. We don't need to say it. He knows how that interaction was for me and knows I didn't eat. He rubs my back and I fall asleep. Sometimes I think his back rubs are better than eating. It reminds me that I am at a higher weight than I have been for a long time.

Over the next week, Kyle shows me the haunts from his childhood. There's Cindy's Cafe, authentic Cuban food embedded within a run-down laundromat. There's an aquarium full of sharks that remind me of Frank from the gym and fish I can smell from the dock. We tour the Key Lime Pie factory and sample sweets. Wafers and key lime tarts, brownies moistened with key lime juice, and ice cream on tiny spoons. I let each sample linger on my tongue and infuse my saliva with the flavor. Then I discreetly spit it into a napkin. Technically, this is disordered.

But what's more important is spending time with Kyle and Lisa. No meal plan. No protocol. No accountability. I tell Rachel to back off, that I want to be normal and she is preventing me from forming connections. I'm finally intuitive eating. I'm mainly living off of sugar-free jello, but also bites of Kyle's food. Rich Cuban sandwiches, juicy steaks, and scrambled egg empanadas, all of which are dutifully spat into a napkin.

Kyle takes me to the gym he frequented in high school. It overlooks the water and has a gritty feel. Poorly working air conditioning, dated posters about heart rate zones and food pyramids, and squeaky ellipticals all take me back to the 1990s. My higher weight gives me more strength, and I see it in the amount of weight I lift. I've escaped into the sounds of T.I.'s *Paper Trail*, needing the world to just be that for an hour. Midset, I see something behind me in the mirror. It's a stadiometer. My heart drops and I know my workout is over.

The seed has been planted.

Ask Kyle to measure your height. You look short. Ask him. Ask him. He will go back to Virginia and then you won't have anyone to take it. If you wait longer than three months you can't get a kyphoplasty to fix your spine. It will be too late. You'll be a hunchback. You'll need to kill yourself all because you were too lazy to ask.

The refrain plays over and over in my mind. I watch Kyle grunt and rack his weight. I don't want to ask him. I don't want to annoy him, to embarrass us both. I would be humiliated to stand in the middle of this sweaty gym and beg Kyle to assist me with a compulsion.

How do I stop this embarrassing gnat buzzing around in my brain, threatening to ruin this day and turn me into a begging, neurotic hypochondriac? The only solution is to temporarily squeeze the fluid out of my spinal discs and invalidate any measurements. I grab a set of twelve pound dumbbells and do an overhead press. Five sets of ten. I get on the elliptical and turn the resistance all the way up until my lungs burn. Not to squeeze any fluid out now, but to drown out the gnats with my own breath, my own screaming lungs. It doesn't work.

Kyle is on his last set, veins popping out of his unmistakably ex-military neck. He's like a German Shepherd, never able to let his guard down, never able to fully trust anyone, insistent on never getting screwed over, never being a sucker. I think I slipped through the cracks, slithered into his soul when his defenses were down, when Joe's death was fresh. I wonder if he would still let me in if we met today. But then I think about him and he's damaged too. We're both damaged and unable to exist with shiny, happy people, so we stay bound together as we swing around in a nihilistic loop. Never moving forward but gazing into each other's eyes as we spin in circles.

Short Bus Shorty

Denial is a funny thing. Not in a "haha" humorous way, but in an ironic, life-ruining, caustic way. I spend the next months of my life trying to lose weight. Not because I want to stay underweight, of course, but because I want that fresh start, that clean slate Rachel warns me not to seek. I restrict and binge, and in return restrict harder and binge harder. This is ongoing background noise as my OCD takes front and center.

First it's the bus. I read a case study on PubMed about a woman who fractured her spine, an osteoporotic 73-year-old sitting on the back of a bus that went over a pothole. Granted, the bus was in a remote village in India, probably careening down a dirt road, and my fear surrounds a charter bus driving down a smooth highway.

This is when my relationship with work sours. Work has always been a reprieve for me, an escape from the demons that haunt me when I enter the threshold of my apartment. Suddenly work and my own demons become one. My poison is now leaking onto another surface of my life. Everywhere I go, there I am.

It isn't my idea to take a field trip. Principal Lutz declares that a trip to the State Capitol is a grand opportunity to bring the classroom to life, and it's decided. I will take a bus for two and a half hours along with fifty students who will witness my meltdown. I replay the video I've saved on my phone, me outside of Leek's house after our final session, reassuring myself that charter buses are fine. I look at my teeth in that video, gray from purging. My teeth are white again. I hadn't seen how bad they looked. Maybe if I had I wouldn't have needed to go to treatment. I don't want that life back.

All Kyle and I talk about for the weeks immediately preceding the trip is buses. "Do any still have leaf spring suspension?" "Should I sit in the center of the bus to eliminate a lever arm, or the front of the bus?" "Should I be over the tires or in front of them?" "What if for some unforeseeable reason I am forced to sit in the back of the bus?" "Is that safe if the bus has air ride suspension?" "Will there be an extra set of wheels on the bus?" "Will this amplify or reduce the vertical forces on my spine?" The wheels in my brain go round and round.

During my planning period, I use the school phone to call bus companies. I no longer grade papers during this time. I call Annett and Candie's Coachworks and Bluebird.

"Hello, this is Pam Parker and I'd like to reserve a bus for my cheerleading team," I tell Terry from Annett. "I have a few questions. Are there bathrooms on the bus?"

These are buffer questions so that Terry will never suspect that I am losing my grip, scared for my spine but more scared that my fear for my spine will keep my esophagus too spasmed to eat, that my fear will choke me and starve me like it has since I was the same age as my students. Terry doesn't know that I have to ask these questions to eat, to survive. I need Terry to help me, and she has no idea just how important she is.

"Annett is the smoothest in the business, Ms. Parker."

I write it down on a post-it: **Air ride suspension. Smoothest in the business. Not like a school bus.**

I read studies. The amplitude of the whole-body vibration on a bus is well below the OSHA limit. Granted, OSHA doesn't know jackshit about osteoporosis, but it still eases my mind and smooths out the jagged edges of my terror. Some days I hit the wall. Every mention of the trip distracts me from my lesson.

"Who can raise their hand and tell me who recommends state tax changes?"

"Ms. Dixon, are we going to see the governor's mansion? On our FIELD TRIP?"

Questions like this hijack my brain, steal the words from my lips, and leave me a babbling, frozen fool. Buses consume my mind. I stop eating at work. It's a waste of food and I've learned that I will binge anyways, lunch or no lunch. I don't have a serious eating disorder though. I just dislike buses.

No matter how many healthy fats I eat, no matter how much weight I gain, I binge almost every day. On the days I can't get ahold of Terry from Annett, I slip out during my lunch period and slink into the Dollar General to buy as many fat-free shortbread cookies as I can cram in my mouth in 25 minutes. Then I return to fourth period, head pounding from the sugar rush, stomach aching, mouth releasing words about supply curves and interest rates and opportunity costs. I look at the faces in the room, the young, innocent, mischievous students who have no idea that my personal life is crumbling in my stomach as I talk about pop quizzes and group presentations.

In the twilight period of optimism immediately post-episode, I always believe with certainty it was the last time. I'm sure that I'll fast the next day, and the comfort of this knowledge is almost as addictive as purging. But within hours reality hits and I realize it's the same addiction as before, but without the purge.

I develop certain superstitions around food. I believe if I follow just the right steps, I won't binge. I don't eat breakfast or lunch. After work I eat my first meal: two cups of diet ice cream and four high-fiber, sugar-free brownies. I'm seasoned enough to know the calorie counts on these diet products are bullshit. The companies count fiber as zero calories when fiber can be up to two calories per gram. Maybe that doesn't matter to people who eat all of these foods in normal portions, but I eat over 200 grams of fiber a day, so the calories add up. Even more bothersome, at all times I am counterintuitively constipated. But it's part of the ritual.

Bags of lettuce and cups of sugar-free jello fill a void if I'm desperate at work. They're the lesser evil. I still haven't had the demon rinsed out of me. But now, instead of wasting away and seeing death as I stare into the toilet, I fear I'll become obese. I gain 17 pounds in less than three months. Rachel tells me it's a normal response, but I can't envision a day where I won't want to binge. I accept that I will never like my body again.

But that's eclipsed by my fear of the bus. If I get on that bus and have a panic attack, my career will be over. I'll be trapped in a coffin on wheels for over two hours while my students and colleagues see me for what I am, a maniac scraping the skin off my neck, cursing nonsensically, and wheezing for air. I wish Kyle could come with me or I could talk to Leeks again. But if I talk to Leeks again, I'll want to ask her so much more than just bus questions. I'll start getting X-rays and purging, and I'll relapse completely.

In an impulsive click of a button, I book a flight to Virginia. I buy bus tickets and Kyle comes with me. We hold hands in Washington Union Station and spend the whole day riding buses. We sit in the front, and in the middle, and in the back. I try out all of the posture-perfect pillows in my duffle bag of dysfunction. It's surprisingly romantic as the Christmas lights glisten, reminiscent of a time before air ride suspension. Of all visits, this one should be tense and full of arguments. But it isn't. I take off my shirt in front of him again, leave the light on, confident that I only repulse myself.

The only dark cloud is the same dilemma that has dragged on for years. Kyle's work is his passion and I can sense his hesitation about moving back to Sanford. He doesn't know if he could ever be happy there or if he would resent me too much. But as we are so adept at doing, we compartmentalize the issue and tuck it in overhead storage with my pillows as we ride the bus.

I embark on the field trip with confidence. My students love seeing the Capitol and make me proud as they conduct a mock trial in the state Supreme Court. My Quest bar never makes it out of my purse. There's no opportunity to surreptitiously devour it as Nancy talks my ear off the entire ride home, but that will make eating later that much sweeter. The trip will be over and I won't have eaten any of my daily allowance yet.

At 7 p.m. we pull into the school parking lot. I lug my bag of pillows to my car, and once the last student is picked up I begin my drive home, hands trembling from the day-long fast. But as I drive, I realize there are no vibrations. The charter bus had vibrations.

Was the bus a rough ride after all? Was it bumpy enough to fracture my spine? The trip is over, but it will never truly be over because the wheels of the bus will forever spin round and round in my mind. I pull over, unable to resist the urge to scour Google. I sit on the shoulder of the road for hours as I scour the internet for answers to questions only I am asking. **What are the**

effects of whole-body vibration on the spine? *What are the OSHA limits again? Does vertical versus horizontal amplitude matter?* **Which is worse, high amplitude-low frequency or low amplitude-high frequency?**

For the first time in the four months since I've been home from treatment, I spit up ice cream outside of the ice cream store. I stay erect the whole time, but as I drive away I contract my stomach muscles and bring the ice cream back up into the cup. Fuck. Technically that is purging. It's a bubble gum version of purging, the marijuana of drugs. *If I purge and I'm still sitting up straight, could I hurt myself? Do I need another X-ray?* No, that's silly. I've been purging ice cream since I was twelve. My body is made to purge ice cream. Or "spit up." Semantics.

I'm floating through life. I seldomly sleep longer than four hours, and after a long day of travel I'm too wound up to even try. My meals are all over, my sleep is all over. So I go to the gym and pick a treadmill. I wonder how far I can walk at a 15% incline. I decide to walk until my mind is clear. I walk and walk but clarity never comes.

Mind Is Playin' Tricks On Me

I never look quite right to myself, but my weight settles around 103 by Christmas. I hate it. I hate not seeing veins in my arms. I hate having to flex until I strain a muscle to see my bottom two abs. The top four are blurry too, and my thighs jiggle when I drive. It's all I see in the rearview mirror, which is permanently tilted askew from my body checks.

But I never lose faith that I'll lose the weight. I reread *Wasted* by Marya Hornbacher and start consciously allowing myself to dip into that world of darkness. I've never found the glamor that anorexia promised me, but I can't stop searching. It must exist.

Rachel has a young patient with Asperger's and anorexia. She wants me to come in, to testify and be a success story for inpatient treatment. The girl is an adorable little creature in a

Christmas sweater. I wonder if she will become a monster one day. I need to be an adult. It's not too late for her. It's too late for me but she can be saved. I wear my favorite outfit, a brown pea coat and Hollister jeans. I don't look sick at all. I look well enough to talk to this little girl with thick black glasses and tell her that Arizona saved my life. I will lie in a heartbeat for this child to not be me one day. I want to be what Rachel sees in me during this time, to hide from her what I already know. I am in the eye of the storm, and I'm about to get sucked up in a vortex and swept away from my sanity.

When school resumes for the second semester, I take my students to the computer lab to create a presentation about personal finance. The students love to show off their work, and seeing their enthusiasm reignites my passion for teaching. It's only my third year in the classroom and I'm already runner-up for teacher of the year. I'm respected here, and parents often request to have their kids switched to my class. I'm more than my eating disorder.

By day three of the project, most students are almost finished. They don't need as much help, and my mind begins to wander. I'm bored. I need an interactive lesson, one where I can jump around at the front of the room, rotating students to station after station, drowning out the voices in my head.

Nobody would know if I looked up the latest data on osteoporosis. I can't. No.

I won't look on Google but my hip is right here. My rib is right here. I have all I need to perform the pelvis-rib test recommended by the National

Osteoporosis Foundation. Is three fingers or four fingers the normal space between the last rib and the top of the hip? If the space shrinks, I'm shrinking too. My spine is buckling and my intestines will spill out any day, making me look like an alien, a pregnant misshapen freak.

I can't let that happen. If it is happening, I have three months until it heals into a new, deformed position. Three months to get a kyphoplasty or live out the rest of my days, a creature without a basement to live in. If Angela takes a week to return a text, she damn sure isn't going to follow through on her offer to let me be her basement creature.

I know I shouldn't do it. I know I shouldn't check, shouldn't indulge this compulsion surrounded by squirrely eighth graders. As I return to the front of the room, I surrender to the urge to palpate my last rib. I jam my fingers in the space.

What is the acceptable distance? Is it three-and-a-half fingers or four? What exactly is meant by "last rib"? The cartilaginous floating rib, not attached to my sternum at the anterior end? Or the last true rib, rib seven? Is that a crazy question? No. It matters.

The lunch bell rings and I retreat into my closet to check my phone. I have a voicemail from Sanford Family Physicians, my new doctor. It's almost time for my Brivina injection and I worry there's an issue. Unfortunately, today is a faculty luncheon at which my absence will be sorely missed, which means my lunch will not be spent eating. It never is anyways. But I will have to take a plate of pasta with a scoop of sad salad drenched in olive oil. I'll push it around, mushing it between the tines of my fork to create evenly spaced indentations in my Styrofoam plate.

"How is little Emma? Is Ryan moving up to the next level in karate?" I'll do my best to act interested, immersed in a culture that revolves around children. I love students, but only my own. I have never cared too much what Emma and Ryan do in their free time or who needs to pump during her planning period.

I love talking with my colleagues in other settings. I live for Klein's wild stories about when she owned a toy store. I look forward to commiserating about the struggle to corral some of our more difficult students. But I don't understand how people eat with coworkers. *If we don't talk about our sex lives and our bowel schedules, how can food be considered polite conversation?* I watch my colleagues nonchalantly put food in their mouths, grind it up with their teeth, mix it with saliva, and form a bolus that travels to their stomachs and begins a journey through their digestive tracts. *How is this professional?* Then they gush over the flavors, *ooh* and *ahh* and *mmm* embarrassingly, shamefully. An orgy would be less intimate.

As I walk toward the administration building, I smell the greasy abomination catered by Donatello's. My stomach reflexively growls, but I'm morally repulsed. I'm running out of time to retrieve my voicemail before the luncheon begins. I type in the wrong passcode with fat fingers but finally hear it play.

"Hi Jenna, this is Elizabeth from Sanford Family Physicians. I'll be in charge of your Brivina injection. You need to get bloodwork to see if you qualify, with a complete blood count, and we need to check that your kidney levels are normal. Dr. Shay also needs you to get a bone density scan. Give me a call back and we can discuss."

My heart echoes in my eardrums. *Qualify to get the Brivina.* Not only do I not want to get a bone density scan, but I have no control over my bloodwork. Every day I stuff my body full of boiled egg whites and devour heads of lettuce chased with pallets of sugar-free jello.

What if all of the protein makes my blood urea nitrogen high and gives the false impression my kidneys are compromised? What if my bizarre eating disqualifies me from the injection that will keep me from becoming a hunchback? I could try to eat normally for a few days before the bloodwork. I sketch a sample meal plan on my napkin, no longer concerned with keeping up the charade of normalcy.

I pull out my phone. Nineteen percent. The harrowing yellow battery warns me this is no time for my internet compulsions. I log in to my patient portal and look at my bloodwork from last summer. The results were fucked up, my liver enzymes elevated, my potassium too low, my kidney markers sky high. I remind myself I was purging every day back then. I've only purged ice cream since returning from treatment. I'm sure my bloodwork will be better, but I can make it perfect. I'll eat a balanced diet for three straight days. I'll have a can of sardines and pistachios for dinner. I'll have pita bread with almonds and an apple. This is how a normal person eats, right? I can do this.

I glance over at Watson as she gushes about little Ben and munches casually on a small square of lasagna. She's easily 100 pounds overweight, and I wonder what she does in private. Her "relationship with food," a term I've always despised, cannot be healthy. One does not become 300 pounds without something happening in private. *Does she too devour brownies in her car behind the dumpsters of Winn Dixie? Is she going broke, spending it all at the Hardee's drive-through? How does she have time for a husband, for Ben, for doing her makeup so intricately? How can she afford those highlights in her hair if she is spending it all on brownies?*

We must be the same on some level, Watson and me. She wears her baggage around her waist and thighs. She brings another cheesy bite to her mouth and dabs at her chin to remove the trickle of marinara sauce. *Would she cry if she got a hunchback? Does she care that she will never see her abs, even if she loses all the weight? That loose skin hanging down will never allow her to know what she truly looks like? What keeps her up at night? Does she stay up at night or does she sleep?* I imagine her life for a moment, wonder if she cares what she sees in the mirror. I look at her and I'm filled with envy. I seethe with jealousy, furious at her for leisurely eating each bite of lasagna as she exists comfortably in her own skin. Meanwhile I squirm around in a watery, mediocre body that will always be one thing: inadequate.

At the end of the day, I walk to the front office to sign out. Principal Lutz's office is catty-corner from the sign-out sheet, and to my surprise she summons me to the threshold of her door. I immediately scold myself. *Why did I choose to wear bootcut jeans today?* They are never coming back in style. Even if it takes me a month to recover from the trauma of dressing room mirrors, I can't keep hoping week after week they will make a comeback. It astonishes me that even after I let myself go, I can't find a decent pair of professional pants. Now that I have ruled out my weight as the reason I look stupid in dress clothes, now that I have let myself get to a sloppy 103, I must accept that I am just a stupid looking human being.

I slap on a dopey smile and pray if I cross my legs she won't notice my jeans flaring out.

"Jen, how are you?" I try to decipher what she means. It doesn't sound like small talk. I hook my thumbs into my belt loop and wiggle my toes around in my shoes.

"My fifth period is a bit squirrelly but it's coming along," I say, fishing for the correct answer to her loaded question. All I can think about is my ankles swimming in these bootcut jeans. I thought I could hide the ugliness under the tablecloth at the luncheon or behind my podium as I lectured, but right when I need to look my most perfect, I'm exposed.

"I don't mean about work. I wanted to check on you and remind you to be careful of old habits." She staples a stack of papers together. Office secretaries walk back and forth, easily able to hear her words. *This is the heart-to-heart? This is the moment we make a connection and discuss me getting to the other side?*

She doesn't seem to think I've gotten to the other side. *How can she not see how big I am, how totally I've recovered from this eating disorder?* Instead I get a semi-public reminder, a gentle yet impossible-to-decipher statement. I play the words over and over in my mind as I walk back to my classroom. *Be careful of old habits.*

Could she be talking about the luncheon? Me looking at my patient portal, hardly bothering to hide my indifference toward the Italian slop? She certainly can't tell that I have lost weight since I am still puffy beyond belief. And she never knew I purged, so how would she know that I have abstained for months minus that one minor incident with the ice cream? Our heart-to-heart, the most anti-climactic moment of my career, took place with five too many people within earshot and three months too late.

Reflecting back, it's painfully obvious I've been looking for a hero my whole life, someone to sit down beside me in the aftermath of the tornado and help me pick up the broken glass. I let my eating disorder be my hero, rescuing me from OCD so many years ago, and it became my tornado. I spent years waiting for a savior to help me when nobody can clean up the mess except me.

Already disheartened after my interaction with Lutz, I call my doctor back on the commute home. "Do I have to get the bone density scan right now? Could I get it after the Brivina injection?"

Instead of begging for X-rays and scans, now I'm terrified of them. If I get one the urge to get X-ray after X-ray after X-ray will be reignited and I will be back to where I was last summer, starving on my living room floor, listening to Rich Piana's steroidy voice waft over me as I realize I've lost control. A bone density scan is a version of an X-ray, the gateway drug to my addiction.

"Dr. Shay wants a current scan so that we can be sure this is the right course of treatment for you."

Right course of treatment. Right course of treatment. I scribble the words down and draw question marks along the border of the thermal paper, proof of purchase for a McDonald's coffee on the other side. What does she mean? I either take the drug and my bones don't crumble or I don't take it and risk vertebral collapse, the fast track to a hunchback, and before I know it I'm buying my first gun and trying to get up the nerve to pull the trigger, terrified it won't be a kill shot.

Her next words soothe my fears and fill me with hope. "It looks like you're pretty deep into the osteoporotic range, so the scan is more of a formality for your insurance company. What's really important is that you have normal bloodwork."

I take a deep breath and flip the receipt over, polluting the **SM Coffee** ink with smiley faces for my future self, letting her know that the person I was when I was writing this was optimistic.

I take a deep breath and try to rid my stomach of the butterflies flapping against my ribcage. I will be perfect for the next three days. Cantaloupe and sardines and almonds, yogurt and water in normal portion sizes. My bloodwork will be beautiful and then I can return to the sugar-free jello and the Monster Zeros and the massive quantities of egg whites. I am going to do everything in my power to be perfect.

I unlock my front door, take Abby for a quick walk, and take off my work sweater. I take inventory of my body. It doesn't look like the last time I was at 103. I look more like 120. The binges definitely increased my body fat, and the fasts dissolved some of my hard-earned muscle tissue. My veins do not pop out of my arms. The muscle mass I've built over the years sits under my blubber, giving me bulky appendages. I consider not lifting weights any more but my back has to stay strong. And when my arms are skinny they look fat too, the Mayonnaise Effect. My body is unique in that it always looks fat. Maybe fat is the wrong word, but wrong. My body always looks wrong. Maybe I will never like it. The least I can do is scrape off this layer of fat sitting on the surface and obscuring my view.

Three days of perfection is all I need. I can do this. I'll stretch and get some extra papers graded, and if I'm too antsy I can walk until all the stress evaporates. I think about Rachel and how I want to get better, maybe more for her than for me or Kyle. She has been there for me through everything. I can be that person she thinks I've become, as if inpatient washed the sickness right out of me. I smile as I think about the tank top she gave me, undeniably douchey but so fitting: **Drink Coffee. Listen to Gangster Rap. Handle it.**

I can handle this.

When I open my mailbox, a menacing envelope glares back at me. The return address is Aetna, Hartford, Connecticut.

Dear Jenna Dixon,

The following medication has been denied: Brivina. Reason: the member is not post-menopausal.

Sincerely,

Mario Alvarez, MD MPH

This is the insurance company doctor who sealed my coffin. I wonder if he's going home to his family tonight, if he is cheerfully eating meatloaf at the table with his wife and two-and-a-half children, not knowing his decision has rocked my world, turned it upside down, and shoved me on the path to a hunchback. *Did he take the Hippocratic Oath? Does he understand one has to start menstruation to hit menopause?*

I call my mom, but it's as if she's never dealt with insurance. She used to handle all of this and now she acts like she's never heard of an explanation of benefits or a prior authorization. Early signs of dementia are only clear in hindsight.

"How were the kids today, sweetie?"

"They were fine," I say quickly, curtly even.

I haven't eaten all day and I have to start my normal eating plan tomorrow. I'm desperate for answers. I can't eat until I find them.

I call the number on the letter. "Rob" tells me I can submit an appeal.

"How long would that take?"

"It varies. One to two months is typical." Rob sounds like he's doing a Sudoku as he speaks to me.

"But I'm due in three weeks. The medication wears off."

Rob doesn't care. He has no clout, no control over my fate. Dr. Mario Alvarez is finishing his meatloaf, clearing the table with his two children while the half-child finishes his peas. There is no way for me to find him and explain that I will never get meatloaf if he doesn't authorize this shot.

I can't handle the stress of life. I need food to cope. Then I'll go to the gym and just walk. I'll just walk until this goes away and the burden of eating, the stress of a meal dumped onto a pile of bricks, will be lifted.

I know I shouldn't eat at 5:00. If I don't go to bed with a fresh meal in my stomach and feel its weight pressing down, I will not sleep. I will feel the hunger pangs, eye the clock, and lie in bed counting wafers and rice cakes until my alarm bell rings. I'm not so thin my stomach will eat itself, not so thin the hydrochloric acid will erode the walls of my mucosa and dig an ulcer. That was before, and I'm well within the range of health now.

I consider taking a Klonopin. I try not to anymore. It was not a good habit. Not a full-blown addiction, but I don't want to be psychologically dependent on that chalky blue pill again.

I take out a box of veggie burgers and eat them over the sink, too impatient to get a plate or cook all of the ice crystals away. There are four in a box and I usually eat two. At 70 calories a burger, two is a bargain. But four was too much. Next I scarf down a quart of greek yogurt, exposing more and more of the bottom of the tub with each bite. So much for trying to reduce my protein. This protein is poisoning my kidneys, setting me up to fail my blood test, disqualifying me for Brivina. At this point I'm better off purging. It's the only responsible thing to do for my bones.

My plans for salmon and orzo, or cantaloupe and almonds, or whatever the hell balanced people eat, are canceled. I can't do it.

I don't have any ice cream on hand so I need to go to the store, but before I do I purge what I've eaten. Five months of resisting, five months of waking up and realizing it was just a dream, rinsing the cold sweat off in the shower and changing my sheets, all of that is literally down the drain, flushed down the toilet.

My guard is down, my armor is gone. I'm knee deep in it, my engine is revved, and I'm on a roller coaster that I can't get off of. I pull my car up to Krystal, run inside, and ask frantically, "Do you all have any corn dogs ready?" This is new territory for me. I have never binged and purged in this apartment. Now I'm right down the block from Krystal, which opens up a new world of possibilities. Corn dogs are a vice of mine, a passion.

"Five corn dogs and a cherry Slurpee, please."

"That's gonna be five minutes, ma'am," the kid behind the counter mumbles.

Five minutes of binge time feels like five hours, but I need corn dogs. I pace back and forth in the parking lot as I wait for my order.

An attentive Asian woman walks out carrying a grease-bottomed bag. "Would you like any sauces, miss?"

"Yes, please. Ketchup, mustard, and butter. Oh, and do you all have any syrup?"

She raises her eyebrows. I need the moisture, need the lubricant coating to help the food slide down and later back up. Hence my need for ice cream.

In a daze, I drive down the street to Publix. I double park my car at the end of the lot, too scared to park near the other cars even in this state. I won't risk a car accident. I drop my keys as I press the lock button, then accidentally activate my panic alarm. There's vomit on my sneakers, vomit on the bootcut denim jeans, and splatter on the sleeves of the blue jacket I threw on mid-binge. And I don't care.

After I fill my cart with $90 of junk food, I load it onto the belt. I try to swipe my card, but I drop it several times and then enter the wrong PIN. I can't steady my hand. The cashier probably thinks I'm on something. I am. I'm high on adrenaline and my heart is about to jump into the bagging area. No wonder I've been so miserable. I have rediscovered the best feeling in the world. I'm nothing without this in my life. I've become physically fat and emotionally flat.

Rachel will remind me years later that I was not recovered. I expected to feel better in my first year of weight gain and abstinence from purging when this is not a realistic expectation. It's convenient to believe that things will never get better because it means I don't have to try.

The bulimic episode lasts six hours, and afterward I feel an empty calm that lets me sleep like a baby for the first time in months. The next morning I wake up and look at the wrappers and dishes and splatter. *What have I done?* I couldn't have done this. This is what destroys me every single time.

If I had a time machine, I would go back to 5:30 yesterday. I would drive around listening to Freddie Gibbs rap about six-piece hot sauce. I would put Abby in the backseat of my car and take her hiking. This one episode has tainted my recovery. In six hours I re-exposed myself to bending at the waist and stupidly positioned myself into hunchback posture. The compulsion to get an X-ray is reactivated.

I try to make it okay in my head. My knees were bent and I hip-hinged over the toilet. I wasn't carrying weight. I used the Valsalva maneuver, which is nature's weightlifting belt. I examine the evidence that spinal flexion leads to compression fractures. I plug my bone density into a formula that calculates my risk for fracturing a bone, and I try to reassure myself that I can move on. Rachel predictably tells me that I should be more worried about purging. That this is a warning, that I can't relapse because technically I'm not recovered yet.

"I'm not going to have this conversation around bending at the waist, Jen. I don't know anything about posture. What I do know is you have a deadly eating disorder. Until you have been weight restored for a solid year, you are not out of the danger zone. Last summer you almost died."

Rachel has such a strange way of viewing things. Nobody noticed I recovered from my eating disorder. Nobody cared.

The silver lining is that I'm finally back down to 95 pounds, only two pounds away from my goal weight. Then I'll gain weight in a controlled way. My calculations are based off of the maniacal math of an eating disorder, but I don't see it. It's all I know. I convince myself that I'm losing weight for a bigger purpose... so I can have the perfect recovery.

Do I know that I'm fooling myself, and that when I get to 93 there's no way in hell I will voluntarily gain weight up to 100? I must. Once I see my angular face at a lower weight I will fall into my own reflection, a modern-day Narcissus.

I try my best to move on and immerse myself in my job. I want the highest pass rate in the state for my students. Lutz will notice and acknowledge me. She mentioned my high scores in a faculty meeting and it meant more than the bonus, more than the department chair paying me a visit, more than anything. My world is starting to spin, rotating around false idols in my mind. I need something to grab on to in order to stop my free fall.

Kyle and I have a frank conversation about our future. He tells me how torn he is. He hates having to choose between me and his career and he doesn't think he can return without resenting me. He has misled me for months, telling me it's too difficult to find a job in Sanford instead of being honest. I wonder if I would have held onto him if I'd known.

"You promised you would talk to Shawn Murphy. How hard could it be to find a job in Sanford?" He's used to this question.

"When you said you would never leave Sanford, I didn't think you actually meant it. Why won't you move up with me, Jen?"

I've never been able to answer him. Maybe I don't understand it myself. The thought of leaving my hometown terrifies me. Somewhere new it wouldn't matter if my eating disorder caught me by the ankles and pulled me under, filling my lungs with sand. At least in Sanford I matter to people, my staple people. If I try to fly away I'll fall flat on my face, just like last summer. I matter in Sanford. My spiral is a spiral occurring to someone who matters. My spiral doesn't matter in Virginia, my spiral is just an untreated addiction, a senseless but tragically untragic death. Kyle's promise to me to never leave is an insurance policy, a trump card any time this argument arises. I take his words and I rub them back in his face. I never would have let myself fall for him if I'd known it would lead to an indefinite long-distance relationship.

"I told you from the day we started dating that I never wanted to leave Sanford. You told me you would never leave either and then you did. Then you told me you would come back and we would get married, and now you're going back on that too. What the hell do you want, Kyle?"

"You told me you were going to fix your eating disorder, Jen. You said you'd stop purging and fucking around. You said you'd gain weight. Give me something to come back for. When I told you we would get married, I was under the impression you would get better."

The comment stings to hear out loud. *Shouldn't love be unconditional? Shouldn't he accept me for my flaws? Am I so bad, so unlovable?* I realize it's not fair of me. Why should he give up his career when I have done nothing to prove I'll give up my eating disorder?

I hate him for being in my life. "I should have stayed with Jason." These are the only words I can think of that will make him feel the hurt I'm feeling, darts aimed directly at his jugular vein.

Jason was simple, Jason was happy, Jason believed we would work. He thought it wasn't that complex. There were no cobwebs with Jason. Jason and I were twilight conversations about med school, walks around Westside Park with Abby, Tupac movie nights, and awkward hand-holds. Jason thought he wanted me, thought he could marry me, that we would be like his parents. He knew of my anorexia but he never met it. Never saw me break a lamp or throw my plate at the wall because a chicken cutlet looked too thick. Jason was sweet and he was smitten but he did not understand my darkness.

No Vaseline

Despite all the turmoil, Kyle doesn't cancel his visit the following weekend. We've laid our issues bare, but maybe we just need to see each other in person. He arrives late Friday night, pale and exhausted from driving all day after working the night shift. We go to the gym, and after watching him eat a Chipotle burrito, we get home and I prepare my own dinner.

"Where is my Jeep key?" Kyle asks as soon as I sit down.

"No clue," I reply, annoyed at the interruption.

"Well I can't find it. I wonder if I left it at the gym."

He can only gain entrance to the gym as my guest, so I put foil over my veggie burger as it smirks back at me. After a mutually huffy drive, we comb every crevice for his key but it's nowhere to be found. Everything starts moving at double speed as my hunger amplifies, but my futile, desperate loops through the weight room do nothing to locate the key. As we weave through traffic to go home, Kyle lashes out.

"If you weren't such a slob I would know where it was. I know exactly where I put things at home. You leave clutter all over the place. You're so disorganized, Jen. If we're going to live together… look at how much shit is in your car. Now I'm never going to be able to find my key."

Kyle's perception of reality is very biased in his own favor, but he has a point. After the chaos of last weekend and the busyness of the work week, I haven't fully cleaned up from the bingeing and purging. The vomit is what people assume would compose most of the mess, but this is very easy to clean. Crumbs, dirty dishes, and wrappers are the real obstacle.

His rant continues. "You don't have your shit together. You let all of your issues follow you into this new place. It's the nicest place either of us has ever lived and you're ruining it."

"It's not my fault you lost your key, Kyle. I don't lose my keys." It's a weak defense, but it's all I can muster. I skip dinner and we go to bed without speaking.

The next day, aided by the morning sun, he finds his key in the parking lot. It had fallen out of his pocket. It had nothing to do with my housekeeping skills and I want an apology. Kyle never apologizes, even when he's wrong. I know I will never get one.

I try to let it go. We ride around town, me wearing his Cardinals hat, and to my surprise Angela reaches out to invite us to a local bar. It's a rundown hole-in-the-wall with vintage video games around the perimeter. I weigh my options in my head. Alcohol sounds worth it today, even though I was slightly looking forward to my six-egg-white lunch. Kyle and I rush home and get ready in a hurry.

I don't like the way I look so I put on jeans and a flowy tank top. My arms look fat to me, but after seeing them in the mirror I decide it will get better once I start drinking. Angela already sounds sloshed in her texts, but there's no reason we can't catch up. While Kyle showers, I take a couple of shots and decide that today if I cut out all food, I can drink as much hard alcohol as I want.

On the way downtown, Kyle's fuse is short and he's impatient with the gameday traffic. I'm tired of his temper and perpetual road rage. I'm still upset he won't apologize for last night. The vodka starts to hit me but it doesn't feel good. It just makes me hungrier. I regret choosing it over food. Kyle wants to listen to country music and turns off Ace Hood. I wonder if we even have anything in common anymore. Did we go over a speed bump in the middle of Kyle's rant toward the truck that was 'fucking with him?' My OCD finds its topic of choice. My spine has just snapped over a speed bump.

"You weren't going five miles an hour. You were going at least ten and it's because you were on one of your angry tirades. You wrecked my car's shocks and fractured my spine. You're such a hothead. You didn't used to be like this and I'm over it. It's convenient because I'm fucked up, but you hide behind my issues and pretend you don't have any of your own.

I want to get an X-ray. I don't want to go to the bar. I want an X-ray."

Kyle softens. "I've been a little snappy, okay? I haven't been getting much sleep. I'm just tired, but it was really nice of Angela to invite us. You can go home, but I'm going."

I know this is a false threat. But it cuts through my indecision and I'm placated by the partial apology. Even though he's been an asshole, I've been much worse many times.

Before I get out of the car, I reach into my pocket and finger a little blue pill. I was afraid this would happen, that I wouldn't feel buzzed. I'm tired of feeling the world. I take half to magnify the alcohol. Cigarette smoke fills my nostrils as we enter Barcade. The arcade games clink and beep, drowning out the hum of conversation. The bartender has his brown hair tied back in a ponytail as he pours shots for a rowdy group of tailgaters. Angela spots us and flags us over to the other side of the bar.

The tension between her fiancé Jeff and I has lessened over the years. The competition for Angela is over and I'm well aware I lost. That's natural I suppose. You drift toward your significant other as you age and platonic relationships take a backseat. I just never thought it would happen with Angela and me. We have matching tattoos on our asses, for God's sake.

I think back to that day, sitting in a lecture hall my freshman year of college. Angela and I took all the same classes so we could be together all day. Our professor couldn't have been older than 25 and thought running shorts counted as professional dress. Statistics 2. I didn't listen to one lecture. I spent my time mapping out dinner, making grocery lists, tabulating calories along the border of my paper.

Next to an equation calculating the calories in a gram of zucchini, I drew a little cat. I passed my paper to Angela. She gave the cat frizzy hair piled high on its head in a thick, curly clump. She passed it back and I drew eyebrows fixated in an expression of surprise and anger. We began to snicker, trying not to look at each other or the cat. Then, never one to let a joke die until it's beyond resuscitation, I added big floppy boobs. Our snickers turned into uproarious laughter, embers that grew into giant flames beyond our control. Our only option was to leave, unable to regain our composure long enough to make it to the door. We stumbled into Kensington Plaza and cackled all the way home.

Angela got her heart broken by some guy soon after and was despondent for weeks. She laid in bed drinking too much wine, mourning the loss of what would never be.

"Nothing exciting or good ever happens to me, Jen."

"Want to bet? If we go right now I will get Cat Girl tattooed on my butt cheek. I swear I will. Nobody with a boring life does that. We can get matching tattoos."

And we did. To this day Angela and I have Cat Girl, floppy boobs and angry eyes, discreetly decorating our right butt cheeks, never showing unless we want it to.

Jeff may have replaced me, but a bond that strong can't die out. Plus, I think Jeff likes me in spite of himself. He's beginning to see that it's not a competition.

Kyle doesn't trust Jeff ever since he set me up with Mosi. Kyle and I were broken up, but it didn't make it any better in his eyes. I liked Mosi, sweet and mild-mannered. We had spent enough time together to become friends over the years until the night we fucked in Angela's bed, Drake crooning in the background. I don't remember the sex. Sex never feels good the first time with somebody. But this knowledge kills Kyle to this day, confirming his suspicion that I'm a loose cannon ready to fall in bed with anyone the second life gets hectic.

That's not the only reason Kyle doesn't care for Jeff. Jeff needs a babysitter when he drinks, and too many times that babysitter has been Kyle. Jeff doesn't like hunting and camping. Jeff was in a fraternity and has an Instagram. Jeff is not Kyle's type. It's a big deal that Kyle has agreed to come out tonight.

I like Jeff, and after two more shots and half a Klonopin, I want to connect. I want to let my guard down and tell him it's all good between us, that my issues aren't a factor anymore. I've got it handled. Angela will never need to watch me get in the back of a cop car again, never need to watch me twitch and writhe on the floor after too many Klonopin, too many sleeping pills, too much fun. I'll never trigger her with my body. I had an issue and I went to Arizona and I got it taken care of. I want Jeff to know why I've been such a mess all these years.

We all do a round of Fireball, all four of us. Angela and I play a shooter game, our plastic guns firing lasers at the pixels. I tell her about my mom, how she's losing the battle with Alzheimer's. She tells me how scared she is that Jeff will get cold feet before their wedding. We go back to the bar. Another shot of Fireball. My dopamine surges. It's the Klonopin. I finger the other half in my pocket and wash it down with another round.

"Fireball!" We yell it in unison before we bring the glasses to our lips.

Jeff and I stand next to the pinball machine and have a sloppy heart-to-heart. Jeff tells me he's going to an OCD conference in Colorado. He's bringing his stepmom and making a vacation out of it. He's decided not to be ashamed of his diagnosis and I shouldn't be either. It makes me want to be his friend even more. We're hanging on each other in a mixture of camaraderie and need for balance.

I tell him the root fear at the bottom of it all, the hunchback fear. It feels so good to finally tell this person why I've been so strange all these years, why I can't just eat. If he knows the reason, it will be easier for him to understand me. I want to be understood for once. After the words escape my lips, dangling in the air between us, mingling with the smoke, my momentary relief is instantly replaced with regret. Jeff is not careful with his words. He's the type of person to jokingly tell me I have a hunchback. I should never have given him that much power, a way he could control me with four words. *You. Have. A. Hunchback.*

Now more than ever it's important Jeff and I are on good terms. We take another shot. I'm stumbling. Maybe if we drink enough, he'll forget. Maybe I don't want him to forget. Kyle and Angela are talking closely. I flash back to the afternoon I discovered their secret texts, nursing their hurt and jealousy at my expense. Never romantic, just caustic and bitter. **Bony little boy. Monkey.** The words are emblazoned in my memory.

"I have to pee," Jeff says. I follow him into the bathroom and talk to him about how cool it is that we have finally realized how much we have in common. I start to ask him if maybe we can forget that one thing I said out there. I want him to forget about the hunchback. I'm on the ground and I don't want to get up. I can't get up. Kyle opens the door to the bathroom. I'm being escorted out. Apparently to pee Jeff had to pull down his pants. Angela covers her face. I try to wipe the Vaseline off of my eyeballs as Kyle stalks toward me and shoves my wallet into my hand. "This is done."

Angela is perplexed. "What's his problem? He's crazy," she says.

Jeff staggers over. "What happened, did Kyle leave?"

I blink at the Vaseline. We have broken up so many times but this is different. Could I have come on to Jeff? Angela and Jeff and I are walking. We're getting a cab and stumbling out of it, up the walkway. Someone helps right me. Did I fall all the way down or almost fall? If I fell then I fell on my butt. I'm in Angela's parents' bed. Angela tells me it's okay, that I didn't do anything wrong. Kyle had a mental break.

The room spins. I feel sick. Did I do something terrible or did something terrible happen to me? More importantly, did I fall on my butt and fracture my spine? That's the worst part, that this is all I can focus on even after my universe has disintegrated. I don't even get the luxury of feeling my heart break.

I have surveyed all three parties involved that night, and I will never know the truth about whether Jeff and I were too cozy. Jeff says no. Angela says no. Kyle insists I was, that I kissed him. Perhaps the most painful part is that it had the most adverse impact of any event in my life and I will never be able to retrieve the information I need to put the pieces together. Klonopin has a funny way of doing that.

Jeff is offended by Kyle's accusations. That is Angela's concern. Kyle has falsely accused Jeff and I have lost the love of my life, any future marriage is over, and all Angela cares about is that Jeff is offended. The big question on everyone else's mind has been answered. But I have a little question and it's morphing, shapeshifting, becoming too large to ignore.

"Angela, did I fall last night?" I try to sound casual, as if this is a minor concern in comparison to the magnitude of Kyle leaving. The thought of falling and not remembering, of having a fractured spine, replaces any other emotion.

"Not that I remember," she says.

I'm hurt I have to Uber home. *If I did nothing wrong and Angela had front row seats to my world imploding, then why am I taking an Uber? I would be there for her.* When I get to my door, the keys are in the lock. Kyle's suitcase is gone, his dog is gone, his Jeep is gone, and my world is over.

But my mind won't allow me to mourn. There's a new trigger, a new pebble lodged in my prefrontal cortex. A backwards fall onto my buttocks. Did it happen or was it a figment of my intoxicated imagination?

Jeff and Angela insist I didn't kiss Jeff. They also don't remember me falling. If I actually did kiss him and they don't remember, it also means I could have easily fallen and they just forgot that too. If they are right and I didn't flirt or hang on Jeff at all, then Kyle is mentally ill and anything he's ever told me, from buses being safe to me being loveable, is false, the unintentional lies of insanity. Worst of all, if I did kiss Angela's fiancé then I'm a disgusting person and deserve the worst. I hate myself. I destroy everything around me, tainting the world, shooting out poison like ink out of an octopus.

I do not feel defeated by this realization. Unlike every other time in my life, becoming a hunchback and committing suicide is not very scary. It has loomed in my mind for ten years. But now there is nothing promising to live for. I click through a slideshow I made my senior year for an English project. Pictures of a happy girl giggling, sitting behind my sister on a tree branch as I squeeze too tightly, posing with my teammates after we won the state championship. I had promise and I ended up a disappointment.

Kyle will never come back. We will never get married, there will be no wedding with me finally free enough to eat a piece of my own cake. I will be a sad spinster. Whatever is going on in my brain, I am sick. I know I'm not right and it's not just an eating disorder. Something else is very wrong with me.

There's nobody I can talk to right now. I need help with these neuroses. I've been so weak. The one thing I'm good at, all that I have left to my name, is anorexia. I want it back and I don't want it to be slow.

I grab my credit card and leave my wallet, still wearing last night's flowy tank top. I speed down Franklin Avenue, making a five minute drive into two, and rush into Publix. I snatch a box of donuts off the shelf and choke them down as I load my cart. Methodically eating and purging consumes the next twelve hours. I chug vodka and dissolve Klonopin tablets at the bottom of the glass, my own adrenaline keeping me awake.

I'm high on the dopamine, and just when my stomach feels like it's about to burst, just when I feel like I did on that crisp fall day, my first day in this new apartment, I walk to the toilet, lean to the left, and close the gap between my last rib and the top of my hip. I press my elbow into my stomach, picturing the cadavers in PT school, slicing through the layers. I wait until I hit just the right spot, flex my muscles in just the right way, and it all comes rushing back out of me. I guzzle soda and ice cream to compulsively rinse out my stomach, only to refill it with the next course.

Entranced, I watch *Everyday Struggle*. Joe Budden is the host and I think of his lyrics, words of addiction and depression that have gotten me through so much. Suddenly his words take on a new meaning. If I have to commit suicide before my intestines spill out, it will all be worth this feeling. I will never give up this part of my life again.

The rest of the weekend is a blur. It's Monday morning at 2 a.m. In five hours I need to leave for work. I can't tell if I'm drunk or not. Purging makes it hard to know. I try to stop myself from beginning another round. *But how will I go eight hours without this feeling? How will I function at work, having to face what I've done as the sun rays pierce my classroom window and I watch the dust dance over my students' heads?* I don't want to stop. I don't want to think about Kyle, or falling, or bending from the waist.

If Kyle and I had stayed home that night, or if the double-date had gone as planned, drinking and laughing with friends, I feel confident that there would have been another rationalization to start bingeing and purging again. There are many accounts of women, fully recovered from their eating disorders, who go through months, sometimes years, of rapid, chaotic weight gain. I have always looked down on them, judged them for their treason. *They couldn't do it, they got hungry and caved in, they lacked the discipline to stick with it.* I hate this inner monologue because it has ruined my life, filling me with pride for my illness when there's nothing honorable about lacking the courage to face the beast that has been eating me from the inside all my life.

The weeks fly by. There's no word from Kyle. Angela sends me a screenshot of her text to him asking how he could be so hurtful and cruel. I wish she hadn't shared. Kyle cannot be in my life anymore. My weight drops, not as much as I was hoping at first. Ninety-five pounds turns to 93. That's not what I want to look like though. I want to look like how I feel and I feel fucking insane.

I don't want to be half sick. I've been standing on the edge of the cliff for years, never plunging full force, always tied to an anchor as I repel down the side. I don't want the rope any more. I want to plunge down and never come back up. I want to leap off the edge and enjoy the freefall, not worrying about what happens when I reach the ground. There's wisdom at the bottom.

Slippin'

Every day at 2:40 the dismissal bells ring. Students stream out of classrooms like ants flooding out of their castles. Teachers gather in the hallway to talk about their days, desperate for human contact over the age of twelve. I used to be one of those teachers, but not anymore. As soon as the clock hits 3:30, as soon as the minute and hour hand form a ninety-degree angle of beauty, I can walk out the door, get in my car, turn up the heat, and enter into hours of bliss. But the fifty minutes between when the students leave and I can are unbearable.

Many days I search through my trash can to see if a student has thrown food away. Like the day Matthew was waving his ham sandwich around in second period, pretending it was a mouth and making it talk. I gave him the choice. Put it away or throw it away. He plodded over to the waste bin, launched the sandwich in the air, and yelled "Lebron!" as it hit the bottom with a satisfying thud. I tried not to think about it, tried to remind myself how disgusting it would be to dig through the trash later. Students blow their noses and throw away tissues all day. Only an insane person would crave Matthew's sandwich.

But it is now 3:00. My stomach is screaming at me, throwing a temper tantrum. I rummage through my drawers, convinced that if I look hard enough a granola bar will magically appear. I can't resist it any longer. The sandwich is seducing me. I walk across the room and use a pencil to push the tissue and pencil shavings aside. The object of my attraction is revealed. Two fluffy white pieces of Wonder Bread hug a bouquet of honey baked ham nestling a bright orange slice of American cheese. I peel open the flaps of bread. Faint traces of mustard are laced along the inside of the top slice.

If I eat it now I will absorb it before I get home. I need enough food in my stomach to purge properly. And ice cream. Ice cream is a necessity, the only way to properly reach every crevice of my stomach lining. I set the sandwich on my desk and take a whiff. Delicious. I stick out my tongue and lick the ham, let the juices dance with the taste buds on the tip of my tongue. I tear it in half, feeling the bread's supple texture. I can't restrain myself. I take a bite and spit it into a tissue that I slide in my jacket pocket, a treat for when I can finally swallow. 3:07. I slink down the hall to check if there is any communal food in the teacher's lounge. This almost never happens, but each day I compulsively check every drawer and cabinet.

I wander across campus to the cafeteria and pretend to look for a student, a thin excuse to smell the wafting aroma of french toast sticks cooking for the free-breakfast students tomorrow morning. By the time I reach my room again, it's 3:25. I can swallow now. It's kickoff time.

In a frenzy, I spastically cram the sandwich down my throat as if there had been no foreplay at all. I make a beeline for my car, diverting eye contact with Lutz, Klein, anyone who could sabotage my mission with small talk about their water heater going out as I let ham and Wonder Bread reach my small intestine, inundating my body with calories. I crank up my car and blast the heat until my cheeks are red. Eighty-five pound people don't sweat. As hot as my skin may get on the surface, down at my core, in the center of my chest, I am always hypothermic.

The ham sandwich day was back when I had money. Back before I blew it. I knew I was on that path, but I was living by the hour, by the minute.

I can't bear a ten minute drive to the grocery store without shoveling food down my throat. Dairy Queen is my favorite stop to tide me over, and right around the corner from Chestnut. But I have to walk in, not trusting the drive-through to give me Diet Coke. The sugar in regular soda will absorb too quickly, not leaving me time to expel its poison. The glucose will enter my bloodstream and flood me with wasted calories. Then I will become a fat bulimic and absorb 50% just like in the studies. I order three hot dogs, a large onion ring, and a vanilla kid's cone. I break every speed limit known to man barreling into the Publix parking lot.

I'm terrified of getting hit by another car in a parking lot, which would force me to get an X-ray, so I park as far away as possible. Speeding on highways does not bother me. If I'm in a serious accident I will know, and then there will be no indecision. I will get an X-ray and not look like a fool for doing so. But if I am in a bumper-kissing incident, I still must get an X-ray. I understand I will look like a fool, like a nutcase, so at all costs I must never let a bumper kiss mine in a low-speed parking lot collision. I must never allow there to be a scenario where I am uncertain if I have been hit.

I put on my invisibility cloak as I enter the grocery store. It's not ideal. Many former students bag groceries at this particular location, but my body cannot wait one extra minute to drive somewhere else. I unlink a cart from the rest and charge straight for the milk aisle, where I immediately chug a quart of milk to lubricate the hot dogs and onion rings as I head toward the bathroom. I quickly vomit, not bothering to rinse, knowing there is still food I'll need to bring up later. After, I rip open a box of granola bars and devour them one by one as I load my cart.

The necessities are two liters of diet root beer, which has a lower pH to mitigate the damage to my tooth enamel (lest this be misconstrued as a tip, this damage mitigation strategy is analogous to extinguishing a fire with a squirt gun- purging wrecks your teeth no matter what.) I need the fizz to coax the food up. Two gallons of 2% milk (1920 calories) are just thick enough to grab the food and allow me to easily bring it up, but not so thick that it sinks into my small intestine. And of course eight quarts of ice cream (7680 calories.) This is business, the non-negotiables. Without these items there is no binge.

A typical day includes the following, in no particular order:
-2 family-size boxes of Cap'n Crunch Oops All Berries (3900 calories)
-24 soft-baked Publix bakery lemon meringue cookies (3840 calories)
-1 Marie Callender's frozen pumpkin pie (2880 calories)
-1 family-size Stouffer's Meat Lovers Lasagna (1530 calories)
-1 party-size bag of Funyuns (to mix with the Cap'n Crunch) (840 calories)
-1 bag of frozen onion rings (1000 calories)
-1 Tombstone cheese pizza (1360 calories)
-12 bananas (1260 calories)
-1 loaf of cinnamon raisin bread (1400 calories)
-1 jar alfredo sauce (to coat aforementioned cinnamon raisin bread) (770 calories)
-2 boxes angel hair pasta (2400 calories)
-1 bottle sugar-free syrup (to lubricate the pasta) (360 calories)
-20 Sunbeam honey oat granola bars (2400 calories)
-2 dozen eggs (1680 calories)

-1 family-size bag of Cheetos (to give the eggs a friendly crunch) (2560 calories)

-1 large can of baked beans (900 calories)

-1 family-size Birdseye chicken fried rice (1620 calories)

-1 bag of prunes (to mix into previously referenced chicken fried rice) (1300 calories)

-6 Marie Callender's chicken pot pies (3660 calories)

-2 bags of Pepperidge Farm Tahoe White Chocolate Macadamia Nut cookies (2080 calories)

-2 sticks of butter (1600 calories)

Total Calories: 48,940

Were these calories to be absorbed, I would gain 13.9 pounds in one session. Obviously, it is physically impossible to eat this amount of food and not purge many times during the process. But the volume of food entering and exiting my body terrifies me. At 85 pounds, I could potentially gain 16% of my body weight in one night. This knowledge fuels my denial, and though I am wasting away, every night ends in self-disgust and paranoia that I did not adequately rinse out my stomach.

I spend the next nine hours or so, until midnight, eating. Every 45 minutes, when my stomach is so stretched I worry it will burst (rupture is a real risk in this sort of bulimia, a rare but instant death), I pause *Everyday Struggle* or *Rap Critic*, walk to the toilet, and purge. Walk back, press play, and repeat the process.

If this sounds boring, it is about as boring as smoking crack. Yes, the actual movements are plain. I sit down. I put the crack pipe in my mouth. I inhale. Boring. But that doesn't take into account the chemical reactions, the adrenaline and dopamine rush, the starving stomach being filled, emptied, filled. I know that after it's over my stomach will be empty. But five, maybe six times a day, my stomach feels the comforting stretch of food, rich, fatty food, and even if it's only there for 45 minutes before all that's left is hydrochloric acid, these 45 minutes are magical.

The next day as I sit in meetings, I look around the conference table. Klein is my Work Mom. Nothing changes between us during this period of time. When you know somebody as interesting as Klein, it's okay when they do most of the talking. She has lived three lives in one. She tells me about her knitting club and her weekend plans with her bird-watching group. She is trying to lose 20 pounds, but it's on the backburner because she's so busy. She's traveled exotic places and done so many things I will never do, but all I feel is pity for her. She's going home to her wife. They'll go out to dinner and she'll order one entree. Then she'll go home and go to bed. She will never know what true joy is, what it feels like to cram plate after plate of food down and bring it back up; the excitement, the rush, and the wonderful emptiness when it's all over.

This phase, this honeymoon period of reunification with my eating disorder, like anything else must come to an end.

Sundays are the best days. There's no work to get in the way, so I perch on the side of my bed waiting for the clock to hit 6:50. Then I speed off to the supermarket to begin the routine self-destruction, first going through the Krystal drive-through for my standard corn dogs. But this Sunday is different.

I pull up to the window, hands shaking as usual, and give my credit card to Raheem, who can't be more than seventeen years old. They know me here, know when they see my car in the drive-through cameras that it's time to put a fresh batch of corn dogs in the grease vat. I can taste them already.

"Miss, your card didn't go through," he says, never looking up from his phone.

"There must be a mistake," I say. "Try my debit card."

It's quite possible I've maxed out my credit card. I'm too scared to check the balance, too scared to be slapped in the face with reality, so I just avoid it and apply for new cards with worse interest rates. I'm up to three.

I don't have the stomach to look at my finances. It won't make a difference. I'm addicted to food, and no matter what I need to do to get it, I'll get it. Lack of money can't stop a need this strong. I rely on the school board to put the direct deposit in my account every other Friday, cross my fingers, and hope for the best.

"It says insufficient funds." Raheem hands my card back and puts the brown, grease-stained bag on the counter behind him.

Raheem probably still lives at home. He could have been in my classroom three years ago, his baby mustache just filling in. Here I am, a veteran teacher, and I can't pay for five corn dogs. Maybe he thinks I'm just a low-life, a disheveled old woman not too far from the pregnant, leather-skinned prostitute down the block who pushes a shopping cart and holds up a sign that says: **Hungry**. These days, I look closer to 37 than 27. All of the subcutaneous fat in my face is gone and replaced by pronounced nasolabial folds, known to people who don't obsess for hours on how to get rid of them as "smile lines."

"Must be a mistake. I'll call my bank," I say, trying to hide the fact that I'm freaking the fuck out.

I don't call my bank. There's been no mistake and I know it. I spend almost $800 a week on food. I make a teacher's salary, which is admittedly modest, but I also make an extra 20% for teaching a class on the side and tutoring on the weekends. I gave up my planning period and weekends to pay for corn dogs and now even that is not enough. Long term I need a better plan, but my worry is the next five minutes. If I don't get food in my mouth immediately, I'm going to die. I will melt, wash away down the sewer grate, and disappear from life. I'll have to sit at my house and think about how I'm bending from the waist, about how maybe I fell on my buttocks that fateful night at Barcade, about how I've lost Kyle. No, this is not a viable option.

Need money now. I type it into Safari. I see posts on Reddit about money by the next day. That is not now. I need money right now. I look out of my driver-side window. *Could somebody have dropped a ten?* A ten could get me through a couple of hours if I use it at the dollar store.

Once I found $94 in the Target parking lot. That was five years ago, and I know this is wishful thinking. But I need hope. I allow myself to fantasize, and like an old man with a metal detector combing the beach for the ancient coin that will make him a millionaire, I drive into the Publix parking lot and do a quick scan. Not even a dime has been dropped. I see a sign in the strip plaza: **Fast Payday Loans Inc**. I've listened to enough Dave Ramsey to know how bad this is. This is the financial equivalent of mainlining heroin, the option nobody thinks they'll choose. Thankfully, they are closed on Sundays.

I tailgate the truck in front of me back into my apartment complex and grab a few possessions. Oakley sunglasses Kyle left behind. An old Yamaha guitar I never plan on playing. A *Guitar for Dummies* tape I never plan on watching. A bicycle I haven't ridden in over a year. I shove it all into my backseat and trunk, not bothering to use proper body mechanics, not caring, and head to Value Pawn and Jewelry. Apparently, what I thought were my most precious valuables amounts to $70. This might be enough on a Tuesday, but $70 isn't good enough for a Sunday. And so begins the era of all-you-can-eat buffets. My private issue, my dirty little secret, will now be done in public.

What started as an escape becomes a burden. I didn't actually solve any problems and added a whole host of new ones. I was pulled in by the offer of freedom from consequences and my life is now one big consequence. There is no joy after work. I go straight to Ocean Buffet. I avoid eye contact as the waitress ushers me to a booth and I slide my purse full of milk under the table as discreetly as possible. I cringe when I see a mother escort her little girls into the bathroom, knowing they will take eons as I sit in my booth and try to maintain the mind-muscle connection I need to purge. I try to mentally will the Foo Yung Chou not to reach my small intestine and make me instantly obese.

I stare at the wall when the waitress clears my plates and try to squeeze as many hours out of this place as I can. I ignore the sign posted over the hot bar: **Please limit your time to no more than two hours**. I block the world out with headphones as I watch *Everyday Struggle, Rich Piana, Rap Critic,* anything to escape. I can't taste the food anymore. The food is just a tool to stop the hands of my eating disorder from grabbing me around the ankles, trying to claw their way up my torso and curl around my throat.

The first plate is delicious, as any food would be if you starved yourself for months on end. Then it is just a compulsion, a mobius circle. My face begins to fall around this time, 82 pounds. It gets difficult to do this in public, not because I'm embarrassed but because I'm cold. Awkward glances follow me and people avoid looking directly at me as I stand in line at the buffet.

Regular acquaintances, Chris, Short Chris, anyone who once knew me, avert their eyes at the gym. I wonder why I don't look thin. I look like I weigh at least 110 pounds. Maybe people stare at me because it's ninety degrees out and I'm wearing a thick blue coat, always the same one. *Can they not feel how ridiculously cold it is in here? How can anyone exercise in a gym so over-air-conditioned?* It would be inappropriate to work out in a coat if it weren't so frigid. This is why people stare at me, not because an 82-pound girl is lying on the bench press, wrestling with the naked bar as it falls too fast into her chest, willing it back up, admiring the veins jutting out all over her thighs as if she's no different than Rich Piana, just a tad thinner.

One day as I return to my booth at Ocean Buffet, my stomach empty after depositing my last plate into the toilet bowl, there's a note resting on top of my purse. It's written in blue gel pen on two napkins folded together.

I don't want to embarrass you, but my name is Laura. I'm not a perfect person and I do stupid shit sometimes, like maybe writing this. But I know that I could never let it go if I didn't say anything. I may not be perfect, but I do understand and cannot emphasize enough that you are not alone. If you ever want to talk, my number is ___. Life is so difficult and it will continue to be, but there is a strength in you that you are not aware of. I know that such a direct approach may be off-putting, but I really do care deeply. I've been through hell and back more than

one time. If you ever need a listening ear in Sanford I'm here.

I hold my breath to anchor the sobs in my chest as they threaten to escape. Tears fill my eyes and I swallow to clear the lump in my throat. I know I need to finish purging at home. But I can't. I'm exhausted. I can't keep doing this. This is my rock bottom, my wake-up call. It may have taken getting down to 82 pounds, but I'm here. This is my come to Jesus moment where I see the light.

I walk as quickly as I can but the tears trickle down my face. My mouth contorts into an ugly grimace and I clutch for my invisibility cloak. Walk fast, look down, and nobody will see what is happening. I shake uncontrollably, not from emotion, but from the air conditioning in the buffet combined with electrolytes that are tired of being toyed with. After several binges and purges I'm hypothermic, unable to warm myself until I sit in a hot shower for twenty minutes, until my skin is angry and raw.

I sit in the driver's seat and put on my Dollar Tree sunglasses. Once I'm sure nobody can see my eyes, I let myself break. I sob uncontrollably and I can't stop. As soon as I go home and rinse out my stomach, I will start fresh tomorrow. Laura got through to me.

Rock bottom is a fairy tale. It's the man running through the airport, right through security, to grab the girl off the plane, sweep her up in his arms, and confess his undying devotion.

It's the tying of a bow, the neat, uncluttered conclusion to a harrowing decade. It doesn't exist.

I enter Laura's number in my phone and draft a text.

Laura, thank you so much for reaching out to me. To be honest, I do feel alone. Last night I set my phone on my toilet as I purged because I wanted to be able to call 911. I know I'm about to have a heart attack. I don't know why I'm being so honest with you. Maybe because you were so honest with me. I don't think I can get better. I'm pretty sure I'm going to die and I can't stop what I'm doing. Deep down I don't want to stop. I'm lost and I'm scared I'm going to die and I don't want to. I can't talk to anyone anymore. I would love to meet or talk. I want to know how you got better and got past this because I'm in over my head and I'm drowning.

I have so little to lose. My finger hovers in the air over the send button, but I don't have the courage to press it.

I walk into the grocery store and get as much ice cream as I can afford, and I spend the rest of the night rinsing out my stomach. As usual, I shake uncontrollably from the cold. I turn up the thermostat to 83 degrees and it's not enough. I get into the piping hot shower, and even though I try as hard as I can not to allow my spine to flex forward, I sit on the shower floor. Exhausted, I put my head between my knees. I should have hit the send button. In the steamy fog next to my head, I write the word **HELP**. I don't wipe it away and I can see the remnants for weeks.

Demon

What starts as a way to manage my OCD and shut out the world plunges me into a different world, a dark world full of hands. As I walk I can feel them grab me, trying to pull me under the water's surface, and as I lie in the dark I can feel them close in around my throat, cutting off my air until I suffocate. All the guilt I feel about bending at the waist, all the uncertainty about whether I fell on my butt, begins to bloom and morph.

I become paranoid about Kyle. Kyle must hate me and I'm scared he will come back to town to seek revenge. I should note that Kyle has never laid a hand on me or done anything to cause this delusional suspicion. But still, he knows how hypervigilant I am about the way my car rides. We spent a lot of time talking about suspension and shocks and struts.

In my free time I drive to different car places as if I'm doctor shopping. I ask them to test-drive my car with me and tell me if I need to get my struts replaced. I spend an entire afternoon driving over different bumps with Herb from Pep Boys, who also examines every suspension component. In a rare act of mechanic's honesty, he tells me there simply isn't a problem. But every time I get in my car I feel a new rattle, a new sensation of bumps traveling up my spine. I'm convinced Kyle has come back to town, driving all the way from Virginia only to cut my shocks so that I'm riding on rocks, fracturing my spine on my daily commute and not even knowing. Every time I see a Jeep, even if it's not the same color as Kyle's, I spend the afternoon reading about shocks and struts and bumps on Google as I binge and purge.

Angela and I used to have a weekly tradition. We'd rent a scary movie, something terribly low budget like *Human Centipede*, and let our dogs play while we watched. The truth is I hate scary movies. Blood-curdling gore is not a thrill when your real life is a horror show. But I don't have the heart to tell her. This is our thing, and if our relationship means suffering through a scary movie once a week, it's a tiny price to pay.

But something has changed in our relationship. I used to be very open with Angela, sometimes too open. There aren't many people I can talk to, and sometimes I needed to vent and let everything out that was going on in my life. In hindsight, it wasn't fair of me. I spent all week covering up my issues, hiding them from my coworkers, and then I used Angela as my therapist while I wasted my sessions with Rachel being dishonest. I knew Rachel would give it to me straight and tell me what I already knew. I needed to go to treatment.

But suddenly, almost overnight, Angela terrifies me. I don't want to talk to her anymore about my eating disorder. At. All. Every time she sees me her face falls. My knobby knee joints are thicker in circumference than my actual thighs. My elbows point loudly out of my arms and ropy veins cover my entire body to the point where even I am nauseated by them. She's terrified for my life, unable to understand why an intelligent person would let themselves wither away to literal skin and bone. Why I can't beat what she did.

I start wearing baggy clothes around her, hoping that she will stop her comments.

"Jen, it's your face. You can't hide it. Your cheekbones. You're getting that horseface look. It doesn't look right."

I try to tell myself she's jealous, but I know she's not.

"How much do you weigh, Jen? You look so sick." She always asks this.

"What do you mean I look sick? Sick with a hunchback?"

"No, Jen. You don't have a hunchback."

"Do you promise, Angela?"

"Yes. How much do you weigh?"

"I'm not sure."

"What's your plan, Jen? How are you going to get out of this?"

"I don't know. I don't have a plan."

I don't have the courage to tell her my latest excuse, the twisted logic that lets my eating disorder once again bend steel to conform to its agenda. If I skip a day of purging that means the addiction is broken and I need to get an X-ray. If I stay addicted, there's no point getting an X-ray because I'll just do it the next day anyways. That is my reasoning for not fighting, for just letting myself keep purging until I die. Hopelessness lets me off the hook so I can do what's easy and crawl into my own grave.

By this point, I am physically and mentally addicted and also legitimately insane. One day Angela takes me by the shoulders as we walk our dogs through her neighborhood.

"Jen, I think you're going to die. For the first time in my life today, as you walked up my driveway, I looked at you and realized I'm going to lose my best friend to this. You look like you weigh 70 pounds. What is your weight? What is your weight?!"

I know the answer to this question. Seventy-six pounds. What she doesn't know, though, is this is just water fluctuation. As soon as I rehydrate it will come back. I look emaciated, but it's not real. I am not really 76 pounds. I'm too smart to be 76 pounds. At least this is what I tell myself so I don't have to admit I'm one of the stupid anorexics who lost control.

"You're scaring me, Jen."

"Am I scaring you because I have a hunchback?"

Her concern turns to annoyance, then back to concern. "You don't have a hunchback, for the last time. That's so stupid. You are going to die from being 50 pounds! Jesus! What is your plan? How are you going to fix this?"

I always have a plan, but I don't anymore. Once I dip below 80 pounds it even surprises me that I don't drop dead. I start to believe maybe I could do this indefinitely, that my body is just cut out for this lifestyle as long as I don't have a hunchback.

Shortly after our conversation, I text Angela. I don't want to hear her comments. I want to die in peace.

I just need some space to get myself together. I have a plan. I just don't want to talk about my eating disorder anymore, and I can't control myself from asking you about a hunchback. It's too hard to be around you. Let me get myself together and then we can hang out again like old times.

It will be a solid year before Angela and I speak again. Jeff will later tell me this devastated her. The irony. The one person I most wanted back in my life now terrifies me. I block her number for weeks at a time, fearful I'll get a text saying: **You're a hunchback**. Then I unblock it, worried that if she wanted to tell me I was a hunchback, I should know. I switch gyms, so terrified I'll run into her and Jeff, that they will see my body, that they will call me a hunchback.

The gym, once my escape from reality and a place to shine, the remnants of my athletic talent, becomes a compulsion zone. Not exercise compulsion. By the time I drop below 85 pounds, I go through the motions of lifting weights but I'm weak and I know it. But there's a new stadiometer in the locker room that releases psychic pheromones I can't resist. Now I can measure my height every day.

My binge-purge episodes get longer and my tolerance for them increases, as with any drug.

I finish around midnight and drive to the gym. Exercise becomes one of the rare times I'm not freezing in a classroom or staring into a toilet, and I need a place to release the manic adrenaline of starvation. But before I earn the right to put on my headphones and zone out, I have to take my height. Over and over and over again. I develop shoulder impingement (no fat causes every joint to lack lubrication) from reaching behind my head to put the lever on my crown. I spend hours watching videos designed for med school students or nurses, tutorials on taking patient heights.

Should my heels be together? Should the lever sit firmly against my scalp or just graze it? Should I be looking up, down, or straight ahead? Socks or no socks? These thoughts keep me there for hours, performing the ritual again and again. The irony is I'm terrified to see a doctor for fear she'll take my height, but I spend hours every night taking my own height.

"Do you want me to do that for you?" an older woman, still wet from the pool, asks. She probably wants to help, thinks she is being kind.

"No. No thank you," I say quickly. Giving a stranger that much power is out of the question. No, these compulsions are part of a tangled web in a universe only I occupy. Nobody can help me. I'm completely on my own because nobody else understands. Nobody but Rachel, but my brain is too starved to remember anything we talk about. It helps when I'm in session but I can't retain it. I promise myself that as soon as I measure myself at the perfect height, I can work out. And on nights where I'm especially tall, I can have two heads of iceberg lettuce covered in Splenda and ketchup when I get home.

Anosognosia is the state of not knowing you are ill. It's common in Alzheimer's. It's the wizened woman trying to take her keys back, determined she can drive even when she can't remember the word for "car." It's the same woman confusing her husband for her brother, but insisting she is lucid. And thinking her caretaker is her husband's new lover, and trying to kick them both out but failing because she can't bathe herself.

It's also common in anorexia-induced insanity. It's a girl in a puffy blue coat driving down streets and measuring the heights of speed bumps and the depths of potholes. It's being perplexed when the college boy tells her to "eat a sandwich" as she walks out of the pharmacy, and focusing instead on how witty she is when she tells him to "eat a dick." I didn't see it, the neurotic, twitchy creature that made people look away. I didn't see that I'd become hideous, that people instinctively averted their eyes, that old friends darted in the other direction. I wish I had in many respects, but I still want to protect that creature and let her live in her delusions. It's thoughts like these that remind me I am not fully recovered, that this creature still lurks inside of me.

Rachel turns up the heat and insists I see a doctor and check myself into an inpatient facility.

"Why do you want me to see a doctor? If I don't have a hunchback, stop talking about doctors. You're triggering me."

I walk out of many sessions.

"Jen, you hide behind your fear of hunchbacks because you're in denial about your serious eating disorder. You're going to drop dead. You do not belong in outpatient and you're very close to losing the ability to choose inpatient. I'm about to make that choice for you. You have one more week to gain weight. If any doctor examined you and knew your real weight, they'd hospitalize you."

I look her dead in the face, alternating between defiance and hysteria, my emotions labile when I'm not head first in a binge-purge. "Go ahead and do it. I'll just shove BB pellets in my socks and wear ankle weights like I did to see the gynecologist. Dr. Ellington thinks I weigh 90 pounds. I can weigh whatever I want to."

The preparation for that appointment had been excruciating. The edema from the broth and heads of lettuce was painful, and it took over a week for all of the fluid to drain from under my skin. In severe anorexia, sodium and water pool under the surface of the skin for days before the heart can figure out how to reabsorb them, so I'm used to swollen ankles and temporarily cartoonish cheeks.

"Jen, maybe I'll record you saying that and play it for a judge." Sometimes she stays calm, which is maddening. Other times she points her finger at me, her temper escalating but unable to be fully unleashed, considering she's my therapist.

"I'll go to treatment. Just give me until this summer to research places and then I'll go. Just please don't ruin my career." I beg, make promises, buy myself more time. She tightens the rules each week in an attempt to corner me and I try harder to slip around her. I'm convinced that I will stop, that it's a choice, until I lay in bed at night and the hands clutch me in the darkness.

"Start reporting your weight. If you refuse to see a doctor then that's the requirement. Every morning, Jen, and you're going to film yourself eating."

I actually follow this rule. I lie about my weight, claiming that I'm 90 pounds or prefacing my number with a qualifier such as "like." I'm "like 90 pounds," which is code for "I'm 75 pounds." I film myself eating, but I can't keep food down without purging it, so half the time my videos are just clips of me in the middle of a binge-purge. I'm full of shit and she knows it, and I realize she is taking action behind the scenes, preparing legal papers to stop my descent into insanity.

There is no point in me coming for talk therapy because there isn't a rational thought left in my brain. Any reasoning skills or short-term, let alone long-term, memory vanished many pounds ago. We spend an entire hour talking about concepts or big picture ideas, but by the next week it's totally erased from my memory. Most of our time is spent arguing about hunchbacks, her telling me I'm seeking reassurance and deflecting from my eating disorder and me groveling and begging for her to answer my question. "Do I have a hunchback?"

I never thought the elation I felt from bingeing and purging would turn into an obligatory fix, just enough to stop my stomach from hurting for only a moment. My hunger is a pain I never knew existed. There is no high anymore from the metaphorical crack pipe. Now the motions broken down are exactly how it feels. I put the pipe between my lips. I inhale smoke while I'm sitting in my chair. There is no high at all, but if I stop my angry hunger will kill me.

As I binge, I scroll through PubMed and look up potholes and vectors and spinal biomechanics, replay the exercise videos I took for Leeks, and compulsively peel up my carpet to check for mold. I rush to finish so I can drive around town measuring curb heights and speed bumps. My anorexia promised to save me from my OCD and instead they conspired against me. I am insane.

I tell myself I'm just having bad workouts but I have bad workouts for months. Fifteen pound curls become five, fifty pound rows become twenty, and my ability to elevate my heart rate at all is gone. I give up. I promise myself this is temporary, just like the bingeing and purging. I'm obviously still healthy because veins pop out from all over my body. My six-pack is more than visible, leaping out at the mirror but also showing every sinew in my linea alba, the vertical line down my stomach. I analyze my abs searching for hernias. I can see too much, and knowing exactly what is under my skin adds another layer to my body checks. I lift up my shirt and perform a CT scan with my naked eyes.

I don't keep any food in my stomach long enough to absorb it, and when I do try to eat my body blows up as if it's having an allergic reaction. My stomach is so used to accommodating massive volumes that whenever I try to eat a normal meal, it looks pitiful and leads straight into a binge. I'm starving to death, but I'm starving myself with massive quantities of food. Why don't I binge and not purge? Because I want to keep eating all afternoon, not stop after one binge.

Once I reach 75 pounds I get scared. My afternoons in Ocean Buffet are joyless, but I now prefer purging in public places. It seems safer in case I collapse, reassuring me that at least I won't die alone. I'm about to dig into my second plate when a Chinese man, maybe five years older than me, approaches my table.

"Ma'am, can I ask you question?" He strokes his wispy goatee between his thumb and index finger and shifts from one foot to the other as he stares at an AC vent. "Do you throw up the food?"

My cheeks flush and red blotches spread across my neck, but I look back at him indignantly. "No, that's disgusting."

"We had customer say they heard you throw up in bathroom. Not healthy."

Healthy. Healthy. Healthy. This is one of the most shameful moments of my life and I'm hung on this little word, a wad of gum stuck to my brain.

I look at my plate of Egg Poo Chow. "I'm not throwing up. But I don't want to sit here after you just accused me of that. Do I have to pay for this?"

I pretend not to see the waitresses whisper to each other as I slink out to the parking lot, puffy blue jacket still on in the summer heat. But before I drive away, I wonder if I should ask the man what he means by "healthy." *Does he mean that throwing up will hurt my spine? Is he telling me I'm already a hunchback?* I comfort myself by reading online forums like The Bump, full of pregnant women struggling with nausea in their first trimester and throwing up every day. This is all I need to alleviate my anxiety just enough to justify what I'm doing.

I switch to Eagle Dining, the campus dining hall, which is better because there's multiple rooms, unlimited soda, and more bathroom stalls. I worry that my own toilet is too short, that I'm having to bend over too far to purge, so I buy a new toilet riser and a saw and try to hack my way through the plastic to create a contraption with perfect purging angles. I film myself purging and analyze my posture to see if I'm bending my spine. The lower my weight drops, the cloudier my mind becomes until nothing at all makes sense.

I fully accept that I am very near death, terminally anorexic, when I see 73 on the scale. I set my phone atop the toilet tank every time I purge now, assuming it's not a matter of if I collapse, but when. I thought I'd wanted to crash all the way to the bottom but there is no glory to be found. The ground won't even catch me and I just keep falling. But the tiny voice inside my head whispering *this is the last time* helps me justify not checking myself in and fully surrendering. If I try hard enough I can stop this, and I don't need to go to treatment a fourth time to do it.

I do not feel happy or pretty. My teeth are tinted grey and the lines around my eyes and mouth become deep. Not a hint of the biceps remain that used to catch strangers' eyes, and though I can see all of my abs, the jutting ribs around them and the horizontal stripes of my chest bones ensure that this body will never be mistaken for fit.

I want desperately to gain weight but I'm addicted to bingeing and purging. Sleep is a joke, just as much an enigma as having an orgasm on the first date. This is my world for just shy of a year. I stop going to Eagle Dining after one of the leaders of a campus prayer group approaches me as I shovel down pizza.

"Can I ask you something? Can I pray for you?" I pause, take out my headphones.

"Why would I need someone to pray for me?" I ask, momentarily forgetting my circumstances and feeling justified in my offense.

"I would just really like to pray for you."

"Thanks, but that's okay. I don't need that," I say awkwardly. As he walks away, I want to grab him by the wrist and ask if he can get through to God. Maybe he has an in and God will listen to him, because He's ignoring me. But I'm more interested in the pepperoni pizza on my plate, so I resume eating.

Hail Mary

I stay up all night on Fridays. After work I binge and purge. Then I go to the gym, buy more binge food on my way home, and finish purging Saturday around 10 a.m. I clean the apartment, wiping every crevice as I wait for the self-induced Klonopin coma to overpower me. I scrupulously clean after every episode so that my body is not found in a pigsty.

I know that I didn't absorb many of the calories and that I need to gain weight, but it doesn't stop the voice from nagging me, so Saturdays I starve. When I'm awake I binge, so I fast forward the day with a few Klonopin and lay incapacitated for hours until they wear off. Sunday I rise from the dead and make my way to the grocery store to do it all over again.

My feelings about death become very ambivalent. I know that I'm doing something every single day that is likely to kill me, but I don't want to die and never stop believing that I'll quit tomorrow.

I always finish my nights in the shower, letting the water wash away what I have just done. One night, I look down at the shriveled body that used to be strong. I wrap a towel around it and get in bed, still sopping wet, and leave a silhouette in the sheets. It officially hits me. I have nothing to lose by calling Kyle. I won't ask for reassurance because nobody can help me anymore. I will probably die soon, and I don't want to die never speaking to him again.

I don't let enough time go by for me to change my mind. I've erased him from my phone but the numbers are imprinted in my memory. I don't expect him to answer, but he does. We talk for three hours, bantering as if there had been no nine month intermission. We don't talk about Barcade. We don't talk about my eating disorder or that I'm now 30 pounds lighter than the last time he saw me. We don't talk about him leaving my keys in the door or me spending months paranoid of his Jeep. We talk about almost everything else in the world.

It will be several months before he sees me in person and knows, before he starts crying and asks if it's his fault. It will be several months before I make him promise not to comment, before I tell him that if he stays with me, I won't be able to stop the daily habit and I'll need him to look the other way. And he'll keep his promise, never meeting eyes with me when he wakes up to pee in the middle of the night and finds me vacantly shoveling plates of food in my mouth.

For the first time in my life, I'm aware that I'm a liar. It makes me want to die more. I don't want Rachel to hate me, and the only way to earn her respect is to gain weight, stop purging, and do the hard work of recovery. Which stopped being an at-home task 10 pounds ago. So I resort to lying. Maybe she won't know. But I carry my demons on my face, in my arms, everywhere. What I do alone in the dark shows up in the light. But I delude myself and hope if I wear just the right outfit or say just the right things, I can have my sickness and normal relationships too. I desperately want to stop now. The fingers of death sink into my flesh when I'm still, so I move until I can't any more. The hours I spend waiting alone with myself until my alarm clock rings are the longest hours of my life, my darkest moments.

I'm parched, dehydrated from days on end of keeping nothing in my stomach but iceberg lettuce. Shriveled from rinsing out my bloodstream over and over again, flooding it with soda and ice cream and bringing it back up, playing a daily game of Russian roulette.

My grandmother was a painter. She never talked about it or made it seem like anything significant. If you met her at a bus stop you would think she had always been a hunched over, bingo-playing old woman engrossed in a large print novel and unable to hear when the bus arrived. But she spent years painting with watercolors and she created beautiful portraits that decorate my walls.

I walk out to the kitchen one night. I need to quench my thirst, so I dump packets of Propel into my shaker bottle and chug, willing my electrolytes to stabilize. I look at my favorite portrait and see Grammy, As-Seen-On-TV commercial in the background, patiently creating this masterpiece and then tucking it away like it's a paint-by-number.

The painting is of five boats in a harbor, an ominous sky hanging over them. There are no people, or even birds, but I imagine captains inside the ships, present in their own lives. Not the coward that I've become. I look at the salt water and crave it. I can't quench my thirst and I want to drink the entire harbor, get on a ship, and sail away.

I text Rachel. It's the most genuine text I've sent in months. **I don't want to be doing this every day. I want to be at the beach. I don't want to be trapped inside messing up every day any more.**

She replies. **The beach is so much better than what you're doing. Life can be so much better. We will go to the beach.**

And we do go to the beach. It's the only thing I look forward to for weeks. I can't stop bingeing and purging, but I bring a granola bar to work and eat it during my lunch break, when I know I will soon have the accountability of thirty poorly behaved eighth graders. I don't want Rachel to see me in a bathing suit, not like this. I want her to see the real person she used to practice restaurant meals with. A person with anorexia, but not so severe that's all anyone sees. Now I'm an anorexic. There is no person.

We plan our trip to coincide with the total solar eclipse of 2017. The moon will entirely block out the sun for two minutes and forty seconds, pausing the world just long enough for us all to catch up. It only happens once a century, and if there's any time to be reborn it's today. I pick Rachel up, still too scared to ride in any car but my own. We don't talk about my eating disorder on this day. I don't remember what we talk about. But when it's lunchtime I know that I will eat, and I do.

We order hamburgers in the McDonald's drive-through and we sit together in my car, and for some reason I don't feel anxious. I feel like this is the start of something new, a new beginning.

"See Jen, this is normal. Isn't this better than throwing up everything you eat?"

It is, but it's difficult to eat just once, to have the food only last for ten minutes when I need to keep eating forever to shut my hunger up.

But today there's something better than eating, and that is being with Rachel as a real person. We get to her parents' beach house and spend a few hours sitting on the shore, talking about teaching and nieces and nephews and life. I tried to secure glasses for the solar eclipse, but my money for them was blown on food, which is not a problem considering Rachel's dad stares straight into the sun. I feel real on this day. I forget that I'm 73 pounds and forget that I'm wearing it all over my face and body. For the first time in months I decide life is worth it and that I want to live no matter how hard it is.

As we drive back into town, Rachel and I talk about me again, about what I need to expect later after eating a hamburger for lunch. My eyes drift to the clock. By 4 p.m. I'm almost always bingeing and purging, but today is my day of rebirth, of starting over.

"Jen, we need to make sure you're safe when we get you home. You can't undo all the progress today. We're going to buy your dinner food together. I'll go in the store with you so that you're not at risk after you drop me off."

I'm touched that she cares this much. But by the time we are back within the city limits of Sanford my hands tremble and my mouth salivates. My tongue begs to be doused with extreme flavors. One dinner won't suffice and I know it. Eating will just make it worse and I'll go to bed clutching my stomach in pain. My stomach will know there is food around and whine like a dog, quietly at first, until it sinks its teeth into my throat, aggressively demanding that I binge. A drop of water to somebody in the final stages of dehydration is the cruelest gift.

I don't want to ruin this day so I try to convince myself I can resist. Rachel comes into the store with me. We pick out yogurt, cantaloupe, beef jerky, and a few other items that we decide would be a proper dinner. But as she gets out of my car and into her own, I know what I will do. I return all of the food, use the cash to buy binge food, and I spend the entire night of the solar eclipse doing the exact same thing I've done for nine straight months, 270 days.

I attended an education seminar several months ago. The guest speaker was a handsome man, well-dressed in a navy suit, cufflinks, and freshly polished shoes that were a bit too shiny to trust him. The story was convenient to tell at a teacher workshop, but the message rang true. He had once been a troubled teen caught up in gang life. Combined with drug abuse, he decided to give up. During his darkest hour, he stood alone in his room, gun in hand, and tried to convince himself to pull the trigger.

Suddenly the words of his first grade teacher echoed in his ears. Every day of first grade, he took out his anger on the desk, the students around him, or, as is all too common, his teacher. She would take him into the hallway after his explosions and hold him as he clenched his fists and cried. Instead of yelling at him, she would take him close to her body and tell him to just breathe. "Just breathe." Those words fell on deaf ears for twenty years as he robbed stores, stole cars, and sold drugs. But they resurfaced in this pivotal moment when he needed them most. He dropped the gun, dropped to his knees, and he just breathed. It took him twenty years to understand.

The day Rachel and I went to the beach, I didn't yet know how to put together the pieces of our conversations or even our experience. I was too far gone. But looking into the ocean, and more importantly looking at a family enjoying life, was a light in the middle of an onyx year. It planted a seed in my mind I wouldn't have the courage or capacity to access for many months. It was a reminder there was a real world bigger than my disorder. I didn't yet know how to use this reminder, but I kept it in my pocket until I finally was ready.

One More Chance

"**I**'ll start eating today. Just give me one more week."

"What's your weight, Jen? I don't want to talk about your bones. Your bones are not the issue. You have a raging eating disorder. It's killing you; it's ruining you financially, physically, and worst of all you are permanently damaging your brain. You are going to die."

I purposely blur my eyes and gaze out Rachel's window at the balcony that overlooks the village center. I can transport myself to a different realm, away from these words, as I float above the shops and salons and into the atmosphere.

"Jen, until you refeed, there is no point in us talking. You need to buy Ensures and drink them. Every day. Multiple times a day."

At times I nod and limply agree, my body levitating into the ozone. Other times I'm combative. I scream at her that my spine is the issue, there's a rattle in my car, I don't know whether the call from the IRS is a scam or not.

I'm fortunate that I trigger something in her to make her care enough to scream at me, to attempt to cut through my eating disorder and reach the person inside, to wake that person up and save her life. She never forgot there was a real person inside of me, even when all she could see was a quivering carcass on her couch.

I am still in denial even once my BMI reaches 13.4. I insist it is water weight and I just need more fluids. I ignore websites that say a BMI below 13.5 leads to organ failure. *This doesn't apply to me, only to really sick girls.* I refuse to tell Rachel my weight. I respect her too much to outright lie, but I can't bring myself to say the hideous number. I am now one of the stupid anorexics I've looked down on my whole life, the ones who let themselves become ugly and emaciated and like they belong on the cover of *STAR* magazine.

I worry about my heart and my insomnia is severe. It's as if my body can sense that sleep is too close to death and that if I slip off I may never return. A once promising runner, I now struggle to climb a flight of stairs. Sometimes when I purge a sharp pain shoots across my chest, and I don't know whether it's from my struggle with the bench press bar the day before or if it's my mitral valve weakening, unable to pump properly. I think back to Frank's warning more than a year and 30 pounds ago, how my heart is a muscle too, and I begin to pray.

Instead of surrendering, I prepare. Not because I want to die but because I think it's inevitable. It becomes vitally important to me to keep things clean. If a filthy, gluttonous vice is what kills me, I at least want my corpse to be found clean. My daily routine becomes more regimented. Leave work. Binge and purge for six hours. Vacuum every room, even if I haven't used it. Mop all hardwood floors. Clean the toilet. Wipe every wall. Clean my shower with bleach. Vacuum out my car and wipe the steering wheel. Go to the gym, measure my height, maybe try to exercise. Perch in my bed for three hours and text with my sister, who lives overseas with a twelve-hour time difference. And repeat. My stomach hurts worse than anything I have ever experienced, the hydrochloric acid caustic in the emptiness. I lie in bed and clutch my stomach and talk to God.

I still have a note in my phone, an impromptu deathbed request written during one of these dark nights. A reminder of the darkness I never want to go back to.

I'm going to die. I know that and I accept it. Please know I didn't kill myself. I fought these demons the best I could but they were too strong. I wasn't too weak. They were too strong. My disease was the most seductive thing I've ever known and it lured me back in day by day, at first bringing me such a rush that by the time I caught it, it was too late. I'm sorry. I love everyone who was with me, even if you didn't quite know what I was going through. And for those of you who did know, I'm so sorry

for what I put you through. I wanted to leave a different mark in this world. Do something special. And I didn't really, but I hope I at least gave you a reason to laugh, a shoulder to cry on, or a person to confide in at some point in my journey. I lived 27 years. That's short but I was, all things and circumstances considered, happy, and I do not regret my 27 years. I am not a tragic story. I'm a short story that ended too soon but was still a great read. I believe in heaven now. Please, whoever takes Abby, don't be sad around her. Play with her and pet her and tell her it's all ok. She needs that. I'm so sorry. I really tried but I can't get out of this quicksand.

Don't Call It A Comeback

"Eat a bag of dicks, Rachel! Ten fucking bags! Suck my motherfucking dick!" Like a phoenix I arose from the ashes. Rachel wouldn't let me die. Like a stubborn cockroach, I crawled out of the quicksand, screaming about dicks and so stuffed with insoluble fiber I couldn't shit for weeks.

I read a story once about a man who thought he won the lottery. He quit his job, told his boss to fuck off, and left himself with no Plan B and no trace of his old life. Then he learned it was a prank, a stupid stunt pulled by people he considered friends, and he had nothing to return to. This was me in reverse. Thinking death was imminent, I acted accordingly. I drained my finances, isolated from my friends, cut contact with my parents, wasted away to nothing... and lived. Rachel would not accept my death wish and forced me to live, forced me to clean up the mess I'd made, and I despised her for it. I was the overdosed drug addict shocked back to life with a freezing cold shower, and Rachel was the icy water. Rachel would not accept my poetic deterioration.

All that I have left is my apartment and my career. Maybe for better, probably for worse, I know that I cannot afford to lose that, cannot let my performance decline. I have no other way to pay for food, no other aspect of my life that separates me from the pregnant woman by the highway with the **Hungry** sign. I overcompensate in that regard, never daring to miss a day of work. I'm absolutely terrified I'll confirm people's suspicions that I'm having "personal problems." Under my three layers of coats, behind an army of four space heaters, and wrapped in a fleece blanket behind my desk, there is a 73-pound body to match the face with jutting cheekbones, swollen salivary glands, and the accentuated smile lines of an emaciated Cheshire cat.

No, they cannot know. I fake a smile, crack an extra joke in every meeting, try to evade eye contact when I do not have the energy to feign sanity. In hindsight, people knew. Everyone knew. But my teaching was on point, my students led the district in test scores, and there truly was nothing the administration could ding me on. Principal Lutz liked me, I think. I hope.

It's easy to pretend you are okay when you are wrapped in the comfort of professionally functional yet personally wrecked addiction. This all changes after one fateful night with Rachel. She's starting to not believe me. Not starting, she's known I'm full of shit for years, but she starts demanding I send a picture of myself eating dinner. She no longer believes that I am trying. I no longer have the benefit of the doubt, which is maddening because I am quitting tomorrow. Every single day she fails to see that today is the last day before my upward spiral. On Last Day #362, I level with her.

I text her: **I'm out of money.**

This is true, I'd maxed out my third credit card earlier that day.

Rachel, I would eat dinner, but I have no money. I will start fresh tomorrow.

You will not start fresh tomorrow. You will eat tonight and you will send me pictures. In fact, I don't believe your pictures.

She's starting to know me too well. I could have easily walked into the store and snapped a picture of myself holding up a Quest bar, claiming credit for food I can't afford and am too scared to eat. But she is on to my ruse.

No, Jen, you will send me a video of you eating dinner. It needs to be filmed from start to finish, and then we can Facetime for half an hour so I know you don't purge it.

How am I supposed to do that, Rachel? I literally have no money :'(

It's true. Until I'm paid tomorrow, I do not have a dollar to my name.

Then you can drive out here and get \$10 or I can call the police to come take you to a treatment center like I should have done months ago!!!

Damn. I'm cornered.

Fine, that's very nice of you. Thank you.

I force my fingers to type out the pleasantry, but I don't think it's very nice of her. Even though I know I have to gain weight, even though I know I lost all this weight bingeing and purging, I still feel guilty. I carry the shame of eating massive quantities of food and there's a little piece to me, or a little piece to my disorder, that capitalizes on that doubt. *Jen, you can't eat again tonight. You already ate \$40 worth of food and this time you absorbed it. Pig. Glutton.*

It's a trick I fall for every time, Charlie Brown kicking the football that Lucy holds up, ironically falling flat on my buttocks.

I drive to Rachel's office and wait in the lobby for her to wrap up her current session. Soft laughter and calm words slip under the door. This is not what my sessions sound like. My sessions sound like Rachel interrogating me, me saying anything to placate her so I can stop the lecture and discuss what I really need help with, which is the pothole I went over on my drive to work. She is too hard on me for keeping these ridiculously high standards that I maintain a weight over 80 pounds.

I think about our last session, her blunt decree. "Jen, I don't give a shit about your career. There is no career if you're dead.

I will call your boss myself and tell her what is happening every day. *Not Lutz!* I will call your dad. I will call your sister. I will get your whole family and your boss on the same fucking phone call and tell them what is going on, that is how serious I am. That is the bottom line. We do not talk about your feelings. We do not talk about your bones. I don't care about your car. I'm not going to sit here and discuss these things with an insane person. You need to be seen by a doctor. You need to go to a nutritionist. You need to be in an inpatient facility. This is not an outpatient-level problem."

I avoid eye contact with the young girl leaving her office, maybe there for a budding eating disorder, maybe for anxiety. Whatever it is, she's held in higher regard than I am. Apparently veteran status counts for nothing. I should be a Corporal right now in RachelLand and I'm still in boot camp.

Still, I'm not a monster and I appreciate the gesture. I know this is the end of the line and I need to go to the store and buy dinner. I take the $10, which isn't even enough to binge with. I fold the two fives, shove them in my pocket, and leave before I say anything I'll later regret.

I sit in my car and stare at the wrinkly green Abe Lincoln. I could have a full meal, a normal-sized meal, but then I run into the same dilemma as always. A normal meal is like pissing in the ocean. Refeeding plans for people at my weight tend to be around 5,000 calories. My eyes want to cry when I look at a well-balanced meal, my stomach preemptively screaming at me, *This is not enough! This will never do!*

Even if I make it so far as to try, as soon as I start eating the world speeds up, the dopamine rushes into my brain, grabs hold of my hand, and yanks me into a binge. Just like that I'll binge with no desire to ever stop, only satisfied if I can keep eating for hours and hours.

I turn on my stereo. Meek Mill. *Oodles of Noodles*. Fitting. I stare at the crinkled bills.

"Abe Lincoln," I say, "you and I are going to visit Mr. Washington at the Dollar Tree tonight." It's not ideal and it's not enough money, but I'll force it to work. I'm amazed at how well I'm functioning through all of this. Rachel doesn't understand that this is the life that I'm meant for.

One trip to the Dollar Tree and three hours later, the money's gone and so is the food. I feel like a monk who snuck out of the monastery to sleep with a hooker. *What am I going to do now?* I'm a victim of my addiction. It's tragic really. I will just tell Rachel what happened and she will see that she has been too hard on me. She will lower her standards to meet me where I'm at, and we can talk about a more moderate approach to my recovery.

Hey Rachel. I messed up. I'm really sorry but I will start tomorrow. I hear the satisfying swish as my text begins its journey. Rachel will be so proud of me, finally ready to start my path to wellness tomorrow as I embrace radical honesty. To my horror, the response is not supportive of my endeavor.

No, Jen. You will eat tonight. Do you mean you spent the money I gave you?

Yes, I respond bravely. You have to respect somebody who's honest.

She's calling now. Against my better instincts, I answer.

"You are unbelievable, un-fucking-believable, Jen. That's it, this is the last straw."

"I'll go to treatment," I lie.

"No, you say you'll go to treatment and nothing will change." She's got a point. "I'm driving over there and I am waiting outside of the store while you buy food. You will eat what you buy and I will go home with you and watch you eat. I don't believe anything that comes out of your mouth anymore. This is over and done. I should have taken you to court months ago."

Enter Jen II. "That 5150 was nothing. Seventy-two hours is nothing. They didn't even make me eat. I was doing pull ups off my bunk bed, hanging out. Go ahead, call the cops."

"Jen, if I call the cops and go before a judge, you will go away for a very long time. Honestly, it's what I should have done months ago, but I wanted to give you a chance to turn this around on your own and not ruin your career. You are eating, either here or in the hospital. That's the bottom line."

I realize that she is probably right. If any doctor in her right mind sees my weight, I'm screwed.

"I'll just manipulate my weight," I say. "I can put on 20 pounds of water weight in a heartbeat." It's true, but ironically this is only because my circulation has become severely compromised.

"Jen, this is over." She's exhausted. It's not her job to babysit me, and to this day I thank God she did. I owe her my life for it, but on this night, in the postprandial twilight of a Dollar Tree binge-purge, I hate her guts.

If you ever see a raccoon caught in a trap, gnawing its leg through to the bone but unable to free itself as it writhes in pain, I want you to imagine approaching it. But you have no gloves, no material to separate you from its teeth. Now imagine reaching into the trap and opening the jaws in an attempt to set the raccoon free. If you have any experience with wildlife, which clearly if I mistake deer feeders for photo booths I do not, you can probably infer that the animal would take out a giant chunk of your forearm, leaving you with rabies and a festering wound. On this night, I was that raccoon and I was rabid.

Dinner goes as one would expect. I insist Rachel not watch me. I do not think she wants to be very close to me as I spew my venom while I watch a bowl of oatmeal rotate around in the microwave. I alternate between hostile outbursts and desperate pleas for mercy. Crocodile tears I do not need to feign stream down my face.

"Fucking-A, Rachel. Come on, man. Don't do this to me. You're going to ruin me. Fuck, I can't eat this food. Fuck man, I already ate tonight. Please. I can't fucking do this. I hate the fuck out of this. I want to die. I want to die. I'm going to stab myself. Fuck, man."

"If you plan on killing yourself, that is all the more reason I should call the police," she says, irritatingly composed.

"Fuck, man. I don't want to kill myself. I never said that. I just meant I want to stab myself because you're fucking with me."

She's not budging. I'm no match for her, and she sees right through me. I stare at her blankly as she gestures for me to sit down at the table. "Find one of your rap shows. What will you be watching?"

"DJ Vlad is interviewing Keefe D about who killed Tupac. It was Baby Lane," I say a bit too chirpily.

"OK, well I'll expect to hear that video play as you eat. No PubMed, no osteoporosis forums, no getting up. Your ass does not leave that chair."

"I can't believe you're doing me like this. This is fucked up. Fucked up shit, Rachel. I can't eat until you stop standing over me."

"Jen, I'm sitting on the couch. I'm literally checking my email across the room."

"Sit the fuck down!" I screech, begging her to sit down when she already is.

"You make no sense, Jen. Start eating. You have two minutes to start or I will call the police."

"Eat a bag of dicks Rachel. Suck my dick. Eat a bag of ten dicks. Ten fucking bags of dicks! Fuck this shit." But I start to eat, truly eat, for the first time in months.

So often girls with eating disorders are portrayed as innocent bystanders, graceful, stoic victims who sweetly cling to their purity. This may be the case for some. But me, I turn into a monster. Years of deprivation and fight-or-flight turn me into a rabid animal lashing out at everyone around me. It's well-accepted knowledge that drug addicts, alcoholics, and sex addicts hurt people on their downward spirals and later must make amends. For some, like myself, eating disorders are no different.

As I write this I am aware I sound like an asshole at many points, but it's only because I was an asshole at many points. I was the anorexic equivalent of a mean drunk, lashing out at those who loved me most, and I'm not going to glamorize it. It shouldn't be glamorized. Any addiction hurts the addict and anyone in their orbit. Eating disorders are tornados destroying everything in their paths and leaving collateral damage that later will need to be repaired. For the next months, I will learn just how difficult the cleanup is.

The following day, Rachel tells me we will meet. And this meeting will not be another hour spent discussing potholes and hunchbacks with empty promises to gain weight.

"You need to be hospitalized. If you refuse to do this, your only other option is to follow a contract. And it's not going to just be us anymore. I want your dad involved."

I don't argue. I am fully confident that I can stop the cycle. Rachel is not.

Rachel punches the numbers on her office phone, putting my dad on speaker.

"Hi Tom, this is Rachel, and I'm sitting here with Jen."

She has told my dad to expect this phone call, and perhaps trying a bit too hard to sound casual, he greets us both. He hasn't questioned me about my yearlong disappearance. I've been calling instead of visiting for the eleven months he and my mom have moved back to town. He doesn't ask, but not because he doesn't care. He doesn't ask because he can't push me away, always letting me set the pace for our adult relationship after the chaos of high school.

I need to speak but give Rachel one last look. I want to jump in the water, but I need her to shove me. She obliges.

"Dad, I need to ask you something." Rachel nods, encouraging me to continue. This was our deal. No more room for my decisions, no more trust until I earn it. "Dad, I need your help managing, like, money..." The words want to come out, but the weekly lies about being tied up for work, banquets, and trips away for the weekend are crumbling around me. I'm naked now, no lies to hide behind.

It was always important to Dad that I learn money management. I was more frugal than my sister growing up, only splurging on model dogs. My dog walking service and lack of spending left me with more money in my bank account as a child than I currently have as an adult. I've never been broke until now, with three maxed out credit cards and thousands of dollars in debt.

I tried to fix the money issues without addressing my binge eating, but it always led to a terrible dilemma. Every extra dollar I made went toward food.

I think back to my final dog walking job, when I realized it was a lost cause. Sugar was a scruffy Maltese who was blind, deaf, and incontinent. My main job was to feed her, mop up the inevitable pee she would dribble on the floor, let her out into the yard for some sunlight, and give her attention while her owner traveled for business.

After an uneventful meet and greet, I reported for my first date with Sugar before work. I didn't mind. I no longer bothered the formality of trying to fall asleep after I finished my marathon purge sessions. I picked up the newspaper on my way inside and set it on the island in the kitchen, then scooped Sugar up. I brought along a scale to weigh her and ensure she wasn't heavy enough to break my spine. I decided 5.6 pounds was well within the safe range. Leeks approved dumbbells and barbells, but I hadn't asked about dogs.

Don't look in their pantry. Don't look in their pantry. Don't look in their pantry.

I let Sugar outside, refilled her dish with kibble, and after ten minutes of tugging on the door to confirm it was locked, I continued my drive to work. This side hustle just might work out. I may be able to pay off at least one of my three credit cards and rebuild some of that credit that has mysteriously tanked over the past year.

The work day dragged by in my drafty classroom, the constant chatter and energy of thirty twelve-year-olds draining me of mine. By the time the clock struck 3:30, I was cursing my date with Sugar. I vowed to make it quick and then start my daily cycle of self-destruction.

Don't look in the pantry. Don't look in the pantry. Don't look in the stainless steel refrigerator I'm sure is full of all the best food...

I set Sugar on a patio chair, wondering if she knew she was outside. I mopped the tile kitchen, soaking up the puddle of pee beside the baby gate. What a shame that this fancy home was now permanently tainted from the stench of urine.

Still, I liked the house. It was modern, and just being there made me feel refreshed. Maybe I could listen to *Hardcore History* and try not to binge and purge today. Maybe I just needed a new environment besides the four walls of my classroom and apartment. Maybe destiny sent me to this house. I needed some dinner ideas though, so I opened up the refrigerator. Damn it.

I thought I was just curious. All I wanted to do was see what normal rich families have for dinner as they talk about their days. Not researching curb heights and vertebrae, but conversing with each other and sharing genuine human interactions.

Interesting. Two thirds of a leftover gluten-free Trader Joe's non-GMO organic keto vegan pizza with goat cheese and caviar-stuffed avocado. Or some shit like that. (If you can't tell by now, I don't know fine, or even normal cuisine very well.)

Next, I opened up the pantry. Sugar was back in my lap in no time, and I don't mean the dog.

By sunset the house looked like it had been ransacked by that pack of wild boars that treed me so many years ago, back for revenge, but this time sabotaging my dog walking side-hustle.

I had perfected my serial killer clean up routine. There was no trace of evidence, not even a crumb. Sugar's owner would never be the wiser, besides maybe smelling bleach. But I had to replace all the food and arrange it perfectly. I gathered the wrappers, laid them on the floor, and made a list of what I needed to repurchase. My penance involved trips to Whole Foods, Mother Earth, Trader Joe's, and several other exorbitantly expensive specialty stores. At the end of the day, my afternoon delight cost me $247, which would only partially be paid for by the $210 I earned from thrice daily visits for a week. I took a hard look at the situation and retired my dog sitting career.

But I don't say this to my dad as I sit in Rachel's office on the Day of Reckoning. "Dad, I'm having money issues."

I don't tell him I have three maxed out credit cards, that I keep getting turned down when I apply for more. I don't tell him I've sat outside various payday loan places, trying to heed Dave Ramsey's advice, but really only resisting the urge because a 45 minute meeting with a loan officer would take too long when I need food NOW.

"Is there any way that you could, like, link our bank accounts? And when I get paid you can take the money out?"

I can hear him putting together the pieces in his mind.

"I just need to not have access to my money. I'm having some issues with ... you know. Like, food. Spending money on it." I look down and realize the pen I've been clutching is in two pieces, the black ink covering my palms. Rachel nods at me approvingly.

She interjects. "Hi, Tom. Thank you so much for your willingness to help. If Jen needs money, she needs to copy me on the text and send a picture of every receipt to match the amount she requested. If there's any discrepancy, Jen knows that we have an agreement."

She looks at me, assertive eyes reminding me that this is not an optional, informal agreement. This is a black and white contract, a legal document. It may not have been drafted by a lawyer, but if I violate it she won't hesitate to hit me with a 5150, a mental hold.

For the next year and a half, my dad is my personal accountant. He dutifully transfers every paycheck out of my account and into his own and doles it out to me in miniscule increments. He never puts a guilt trip on me, never acts irritated or fishes for more information, never brings up the fact I've been ten minutes away for over a year and have only called on the phone. What I don't know is that his hands are full, and that my mom's increasingly rare emails aren't full of typos and word salad because she's in a hurry or bad at typing. Early-onset Alzheimer's is slowly erasing her mind. After a few months, I miss seeing them too much.

"Dad, I want to come over again but I'm scared. Do you promise if I visit, you and Mom won't comment on my weight?"

"Of course not, we never would. You're an adult now. We're always here, Jen."

I'm scared Mom won't be able to control her tongue. I don't yet realize that she will be trying to hide her own dementia from me, using a vacant laugh to mask her inability to understand.

For my first visit with my parents in over a year, I wear two padded bras, my signature silicone butt pads, polyester sweatpants, and a thick black sweatshirt Kyle bought me. It has a pug with gold chains on the front, and it reads: **PUG LIFE**. When he surprised me with it, I was annoyed he wasted money on something so tacky. But now, I reason, an ugly sweatshirt is a genius way to detract attention from myself.

"Dad, there's another thing." I think back to two Christmases ago when my mom playfully clutched the back of my neck and I spent the rest of the night online searching: **vertebral compression fracture** and **cervical spine**, not allowing myself to eat until I'd found enough reassuring information. Which was never.

"I'm really scared of being touched. Is it possible that we can skip the hug?" My fear of hugs is now not just Jason, but everyone.

"Sure, just come on over and we can fist bump instead. No hugs, I promise."

I consider it. A fist bump would be okay. And to this day, Mom has trouble remembering how to open the door, but I can tell every time I walk through it she has rehearsed giving me a fist bump. And she remembers every single time. Maybe it's a blessing she understands less than she used to, at least for the first few months of my refeeding.

"Honey, it's really hot. Aren't you burning up in that sweatsuit?"

"No, I'm comfortable," I lie.

My organs roast in the June heat. The nutrition begins to work, but the carbohydrates dilate every vein in my body and my legs look like two erect penises. My thighs and calves are covered in ugly purple knots. My forearms resemble a bundle of ropes. The bicep vein I'd longed for so long ago is there, but it blends into the roadmap of blue lines from every other vein I have, popping out rudely. I try not to think back to the cadavers in PT school, separating the veins out to trace them with my probe, memorizing the path each one takes back to the heart.

My mom's condition isn't a total surprise. She has asked me the same questions on our weekly phone calls for some time. But it's more striking in person, and it finally sets in that she's gone.

"How are your kids this year? I hope you get really good..." she'll say, unable to find the right word to end her sentence. It doesn't matter if it's summer break or if I've already answered that same question twice in the last ten minutes. She never fails to ask. Seeing her in person makes it final. I quickly push down the sense of relief that she can't comprehend how sick I am.

There will never be any closure with her, no heart-to-heart conversation where I confront her about aspects of my childhood I need to make peace with. The mom who raised me no longer exists. Of course this is sad, but it's also an opportunity to start over and have a new relationship with a new mom. I don't have to be thirty years old carrying around baggage from my childhood. The person who said "fuck you" to my five-year-old self, the person who told me I was getting chubby and who pressured me to wear makeup before I was ready, that person no longer exists. She's been replaced by a simpler mom, a mom I color with, a mom who fumbles with her words, a mom who can't read let alone write an email. It's different and it's difficult and it's life.

Eating makes me furious some days. My coping mechanism, purging, is completely taken away. Klonopin days no longer exist. I can no longer press the fast forward button on my hunger and anxiety and sprawl limply on the couch as I watch the lizards crawl across my window pane. I have to be awake and present in every step of my own resurrection.

I'm accountable for each and every meal and must send Rachel proof. I have no extra money, not even to buy a cup of coffee. I ask my dad to drop specific amounts in my account. Every hour I write a statement that reminds me how serious my eating disorder is and how much denial I am in. Statements like: **I focus on vans and Leeks and measuring angles so**

that I can avoid looking at my eating disorder, which is what will actually kill me.

"Dad, can you drop me $23.26?" This is how exact my money requests must be, because even an extra $5 could be enough to binge and purge. I can't have any food in the house, not even a bottle of mustard, so I go to the grocery store three times a day to buy my next meal. I can't trust myself to eat at home, next to the toilet that has seen so much, so I only eat in public. Inside Subway restaurants, study rooms at the public library, the changing rooms at the gym, and my arctic classroom at work. The lockers at the gym become my pantry, as any food stored at home would be the equivalent of an alcoholic storing beer in his fridge. I have no other place to stash food with multiple servings like boxes of oatmeal.

I'm relieved to be cornered. The contract Rachel and I create is a magical agreement that protects me from my OCD. It gives me permission to not dive into PubMed and drive around measuring curbs. Any compulsive desire I have is written on the contract and promptly banned. If I make a contract and I ban going to the Brivina website for that day, I am safe from myself. The buses and potholes and measuring toilets all are addressed in my contract with Rachel. I can excuse myself from these compulsions because following the rules Rachel and I create is more important, and also the only reason I'm alive.

I'm finally safe from my tyrannical OCD, and this allows me to eat. The only catch is that if I start lying about my food, it makes the contract meaningless and I no longer have protection from my OCD. At least this is what I believe. At 73 pounds I am very superstitious, and it saves my life.

I view lying to Rachel as a pathway into all of the compulsions that make me miserable. I turn a drastic 180 into genuine radical honesty. I tell on myself. If I'm at work and I want to binge and purge, I text Rachel and tell her. The contract is a way to protect me from my OCD and also ensure that I eat, and I follow it like a Bible. When I don't, because I do have slips, I report them.

For the first time in my life, I find a tool that works better than my eating disorder to manage my OCD, and it actually works at the root of the issue instead of being a Band-Aid. Some days I wonder if my life is too good to be true. The ability to eat dinner is indescribably wonderful.

But I also have a terrible temper. Any threat to food pushes me over the edge. An unwanted phone call, a sound in my car, or a pop-up on my computer is enough to send me into a frantic tailspin. I feel anorexia's fingers clutch me again and I blame it on eating. I want so badly to align with my eating disorder so I don't feel as afraid of the fingers grabbing at me, waiting for me to get complacent. I want to feel like they are my fingers and not an evil outside force trying to starve me, because if they are mine they seem less terrifying. But the truth is, starvation is terrifying. Anorexia is terrifying. I realize what an asshat my eating disorder has been for so many years and that it has never been on my side.

My stomach forgot how to digest, and after meals I experience searing stomach pain and heartburn. Sometimes I vomit involuntarily, chunks of food from twelve hours prior coming up still fully intact. Purging is a quick fix, the only way to dull the gnawing and sedate myself. Now that this outlet is gone, I can't teleport out of my body and escape for hours on end. My OCD is untamable, and the only way to get through it is by following the contract Rachel and I make.

I'm aware that I now need to gain almost 30 pounds, and the hunger I feel as I start to eat is an insatiable, desperate cruelty. The minute my body realizes there is food and it will remain in my stomach, it demands more, screaming at me and filling my dreams with vivid images of my teeth sinking into oily hamburgers. If at any time I am not filled to the brim, I enter a state of panic. Rachel calls it "trauma from starvation."

I struggle with unquenchable cravings for food. My appetite only increases when I raise my calories, a common phenomenon in anorexia recovery. A body in the throes of starvation gives up, but once it knows there is access to food again, it demands it. For anorexics who also binge and purge, this is a constant threat.

To tame the urge to binge, I eat unlimited vegetables and sugar-free jello in addition to my meal plan. Carrots are hard to purge, so I once again turn orange. Vegetables become the methadone to binges, and I have to accept that until I stop starving myself I'll be packed full of them. In my first months of "detox," it takes 48 sugar-free jellos, three pounds of carrots, two heads of iceberg lettuce, two whole tomatoes, and a family-size bag of broccoli every day on top of my meal plan. Sometimes in the middle of the night, I wake up in a panic that I'll starve and drive to the store just for carrots. Every time I try to eat more normally before I'm ready, I slip up. I finally have to surrender and trust that weight gain will work. And it does- I haven't touched carrots in months.

I gain the first 20 pounds in four months and I realize how bad I'd looked before. The pictures in my phone make me nauseous. I don't erase them because I don't want to forget. I wasn't different at all from the women on the cover of *STAR* magazine. My invisibility blanket was never real, and for vanity reasons I never want to go back. But that isn't enough. Recovery isn't about wanting it badly enough; it's about making a new decision each and every day to do the work.

Rachel is the only reason I'm alive. There aren't words to say what she did for me. Below is the homemade rap I gave to her that Christmas, the closest I can get to doing this year justice.

Merry Christmas, Rachel T, this year has been so awful
It started bright and cheery with denial and some waffles
But then you screamed me out of my merry manic state
I owe you my life for that, I almost died at twenty-eight
But instead of coming back to life with faith and gratitude
Jen II took my place and gave you so much attitude

You let me borrow money once and in an hour it was blown

You called to help me manage meals and I just hung up the phone

I didn't glide back into life, it was more like a crash landing

I screamed at you to sit down, but the truth is you weren't standing

But you never enabled Jen II, you made me be accountable

Even when I felt like my issues were just too insurmountable

I was swimming laps around a little plastic castle

But through it all you helped me even when I was an asshole

You made me stick to rap when normal thoughts had left my mind

You helped me get through dinner more than Tekashi 69

Though most of my celebrities are not people you adore

I can tell that Ben Affleck could get your clothes on the floor

February I think was when we started the contract

It helped replace the habits, and we kept in close contact

I lost my mind, we fought a lot, but I valued your support

Even when that tough love was you threatening me with court

But I trust who I trust, and with those few friends I stick

Even when there are some moments when I'm yelling "Eat a dick"

~~But I never said that to you,~~ and that shows how much you mean

You've helped me help myself since I was just a troubled teen

Speaking of teens, there's Bandit, and now you have another!

And I'm honored to get to babysit the darling Thompson brothers

And all my issues aside, I'm the luckiest girl alive

To enter into a new year with Abby by my side

When it comes to your new doggies, you know that she approves

Especially when Bandit comes behind her with his moves

I'm not sure where he learned those, but I won't make accusations

Since he isn't neutered yet, Abby must be a temptation

And I'm writing this rhyme early, I'll take it out if it goes bad

But your surgery will be okay, it sucks it makes you sad

Not many people are cool enough to grow their own grapefruits

And I hope you keep it in a jar to show to people just for proof

As I look back on this year, I have regrets for how I've acted

Too many nights under my car, looking for new scratches
Too many days lashing out, or meetings where I've cried
But you helped me get the courage to see the truth and
to survive
So here's to 2019, I won't make a promise or prediction
Because the past decade has been restriction and
addiction
But my goal is to be someone that you and I would like
to know
Thank you for helping me hold on when I wanted to let
go

Changes

As I write this, I'm wrestling with the last five pounds I need to gain. There are five pounds separating me from beginning my mental rehabilitation.

I've sat across from women who have spent a decade wrestling with the same two pounds. Sharon's words echo in my head during my high school dietician sessions. I was too busy trying not to wet her couch to listen, and I regret that to my core. This is now me.

And it's still me. I live with the knowledge that I could drop down to 73 pounds the second I lose insight. My eating disorder is a formidable opponent, and sometimes I get tired treading water when it feels like I'm not getting anywhere. I still can't go to restaurants and have no idea how to eat without a food scale. I sit with my family while they eat dinner and then I go home and eat mine, praying it doesn't explode into a series of compulsions I have to get through before I can take my next bite. I'm traumatized from the nights my oatmeal has grown cold while I measure my toilet or check my car for new scratches that mean I was in an accident. Those nights are the worst nights, when I want to give up and go back to my old ways. But there is no wisdom at the bottom. There is only hard ground. So I will tread water for as long as it takes, even if that means forever, because the second I stop trying my anorexia will pull me beneath the surface and fill my lungs with water. And I will die.

Chronic eating disorders are like viruses. They mutate into variants that evade treatment. Do I feel a daily desire to be thin? To lose weight? No. Frankly, my or anyone else's eating disorder stopped being interesting to me after the initial thrill almost twenty years ago. But by developing an eating disorder at twelve, then failing to seek help or surrender for years, I allowed myself to be raised by anorexia. Now there is a great deal of deprogramming that needs to happen. After years of panic attacks, purges, and explosive fights at meals, my body enters fight-or-flight instinctually. My mind pelts me with thoughts meant to distract me, meant to make me give up and be weak.

I have worms. I forgot to get the mail. Did I turn off the hose? I must order Brivina now. My carpet has mold and it will inactivate my Brivina. What's my tire pressure? Is this mole cancerous?

And I have to sit and eat as I feel the world in flames around me, only to finish and realize there was no fire at all.

Every hour of every day I text Rachel a statement that helps me keep the big picture in mind. Statements about how I have to gain weight to get my brain back, and even on days when my denial is thick and I don't feel at risk, I have to be on alert. I can never let my guard down because my eating disorder lurks around every corner waiting to grab me by the throat and pull me back into its vortex.

I can manage my own money now. My binges and purges are few and far between. But strangely, the second I feel safe from the habit I have a slip. I do not keep a seat on my toilet. It's just a naked bowl. It got so hard to clean every nook and cranny at my worst that I unscrewed the seat and never had enough time between purges to put it back. It's been six months since I purged. I could probably screw it back on. But I won't, because that tells my eating disorder I've let my guard down. I need to feel like I might purge tonight because that is reality. And I'm tired of being in denial.

Kyle and I are indefinitely long distance, but we're happy. Angela and I are friends, but it's not the same. Getting as sick as I did changed the way people see me. I crossed over an invisible threshold and joined the mentally ill side. Not the convenient mental illnesses that can be featured on shows like *Monk*, or where I can say "I'm so OCD." No, the kind of mental illness that makes people uncomfortable. The kind you still can't talk about during Mental Health Awareness Month.

What looks rigid to other people is actually me in my recovery. I can no longer skip steps or believe in a quick fix. I can't ever have another trip to the Keys where I choose bonding with Kyle and his mom over eating a plate of food. These are behaviors that look healthy on the outside, like I'm being flexible, but lead to a relapse. I worry that I'm doomed to a life of 70% recovery, but as Rachel reminds me, I don't have the right to make that judgement until I have been 100 pounds for six months. Then I can decide if recovery is worth it.

On the surface I feel like I've been in recovery since I was sixteen, but I've been in my own version of recovery. I've tried to avoid the inevitable weight that I need to gain to heal my brain. Now there's a bigger mess to clean up because of all the neural pathways I have built around eating disorder behaviors. I allowed my issues to multiply as I tried essential oils, meditation, and other convenient remedies when weight gain is the only chemotherapy powerful enough to destroy the malignancy of an eating disorder. I hope that it's possible for me to be 100% recovered, but even if it isn't, I don't have a choice. I have to keep trying, because the second I stop I will be 0% recovered and I will die.

If I claimed I've gotten to the other side, I would surely relapse immediately. I'm still me, with all of my issues. But knowing that gives me a chance to one day be a better me, and that's what will keep me treading water for as long as it takes. A smart person learns from their mistakes. A wise person learns from the mistakes of others. So though this is not a self-help book in any way, shape or form, I hope the wisdom I gleaned from my journey saves someone else sixteen years of their own life. Take it from me. There's no glamor in starvation and there's no wisdom at the bottom.

Thank you so much for joining me! If you enjoyed the read, please help other readers find my book by leaving a quick review.

About the Author

Jen Dixon is an educator, mentor to at-risk youth, and mental health advocate. She is a published poet and enjoys writing (but not performing!) raps. In her free time she enjoys getting lost in nature, spending time with family, and fostering dogs-though in the end she adopts every single one. She values anonymity when she is not publishing tell-all memoirs. For a less flattering bio, start at page one.

26541450R00215